CW00923397

Ambient Integrated Robotics

The Cambridge Handbooks in Construction Robotics series gives professionals, researchers, lecturers, and students basic conceptual and technical skills and strategies to manage, research, or teach the implementation of advanced automation and robot-technology-based processes and technologies in construction. The books discuss progress in robot systems theory and demonstrate their integration using real systematic applications and projections.

The new research field of Ambient/Active Assisted Living (AAL) is quickly evolving. *Ambient Integrated Robotics* provides an easy-to-understand medical perspective to architects, designers, and engineers, bridging the different disciplines and showing how they fuse together to create the future of AAL technology. Using robotics as an example, the book illustrates how embedding its subsystems results in unique ambient technology that can be used to help people, particularly in adapting to the needs of ailing and aging populations. You will walk away with the knowledge and tools to contribute to the future of AAL.

Thomas Bock is a professor of building realization and robotics at the Technical University of Munich. He is a member of several boards of directors of international associations and of several international academies in Europe, the Americas, and Asia. Professor Bock serves on several editorial boards, heads various working commissions and groups of international research organizations, and has authored and co-authored books from the Cambridge Handbooks in Construction Robotics series and about 500 articles.

Thomas Linner is a research associate in building realization and robotics at the Technical University of Munich. He is a specialist in the area of automated production of building products as well as in the enhancement of the performance of building products by advanced technology. Dr. Linner has received several prizes and grants, including a Japanese Center of Excellence Grant for research in Japan.

Jörg Güttler is a research associate, Chair for Building Realization and Robotics, at the Technical University of Munich. His research interests are in AAL, health monitoring, disease prevention, embedded sensors, medical devices, wearable robotics, and human–machine interfaces.

Kepa Iturralde is a research associate, Chair for Building Realization and Robotics, at the Technical University of Munich. He is focused on developing robotic, automation, and digital manufacturing technology into building renovation.

Ambient Integrated Robotics

Automation and Robotic Technologies for Maintenance, Assistance, and Service

THOMAS BOCK
Technical University of Munich

THOMAS LINNER
Technical University of Munich

JÖRG GÜTTLER
Technical University of Munich

KEPA ITURRALDE
Technical University of Munich

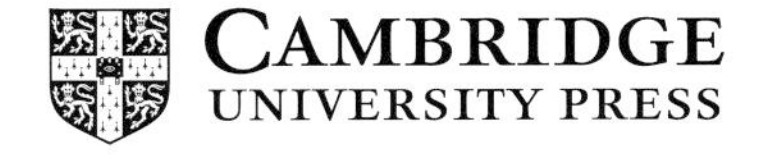

CAMBRIDGE
UNIVERSITY PRESS

University Printing House, Cambridge CB2 8BS, United Kingdom

One Liberty Plaza, 20th Floor, New York, NY 10006, USA

477 Williamstown Road, Port Melbourne, VIC 3207, Australia

314–321, 3rd Floor, Plot 3, Splendor Forum, Jasola District Centre, New Delhi – 110025, India

79 Anson Road, #06–04/06, Singapore 079906

Cambridge University Press is part of the University of Cambridge.

It furthers the University's mission by disseminating knowledge in the pursuit of
education, learning, and research at the highest international levels of excellence.

www.cambridge.org
Information on this title: www.cambridge.org/9781107075986
DOI: 10.1017/9781139872034

© Thomas Bock, Thomas Linner, Kepa Iturralde, and Jörg Güttler 2019

This publication is in copyright. Subject to statutory exception
and to the provisions of relevant collective licensing agreements,
no reproduction of any part may take place without the written
permission of Cambridge University Press.

First published 2019

Printed in Singapore by Markono Print Media Pte Ltd

A catalogue record for this publication is available from the British Library.

Library of Congress Cataloging-in-Publication Data
Names: Bock, Thomas, 1957– author.
Title: Ambient integrated robotics : automation and robotic technologies for maintenance, assistance, and service / Thomas Bock, Technische Universität München, Thomas Linner, Technische Universität München, Jörg Güttler, Technische Universität München, Kepa Iturralde, Technische Universität München.
Description: New York : Cambridge University Press, 2019. | Series: The Cambridge handbooks on construction robotics series ; volume 5 | Includes bibliographical references and index.
Identifiers: LCCN 2018060439 | ISBN 9781107075986 (hardback)
Subjects: LCSH: Self-help devices for older people. | Assistive computer technology. | Ambient intelligence. | Robotics–Human factors. | BISAC: TECHNOLOGY & ENGINEERING / Engineering (General).
Classification: LCC HV1569.5 .B59 2019 | DDC 681/.761–dc23
LC record available at https://lccn.loc.gov/2018060439

ISBN 978-1-107-07598-6 Hardback

Cambridge University Press has no responsibility for the persistence or accuracy
of URLs for external or third-party internet websites referred to in this publication
and does not guarantee that any content on such websites is, or will remain,
accurate or appropriate.

Contents

Acknowledgments

The authors would like to express their deepest gratitude to Prof. Dr. Yositika Utida, as well as to Prof. Dr. Yujiro Shinoda. In addition, the authors would like to thank the Japan Science Society, for sponsoring the initial research on "Life Support System in an aging Society" between 1985 and 1988. Further we are grateful to Dr.-Ing. Christos Georgoulas for his support in writing this book, as well as for his involvement in the development of different prototypes described in the book. Furthermore, the authors would like to thank Mr. Andreas Bittner for his support in developing several prototypes, which are described in this book. Additionally, the authors would like to thank the Consortia of LISA-Habitec for providing the mock-up as base for some prototypes, which are presented in this book. In addition, the authors would like to thank Mr. Ben Toornstra for his support in Chapter 3 and Dr. Y. Suematsu from the Nagoya University for his valuable input regarding the Karakuris. For the support in preparing different images depicted in this book the authors would like to thank Mr. Wen Pan, Mr. Dany Bassily, Mr. Rushab Saha, Mr. Alex Liu Cheng, and Mr. Bogdan Gerogescu. For contributing valuable knowledge at Chapter 3 the authors would like to express their gratitude to Mr. Rongbo Hu and Mr. Wen Pan. Also, we acknowledge Mr. Helal and especially Mr. Schlandt for his effort preparing the images in this book.

The LISA Habitec Consortia consists of the following companies: MM Design, Pfeifer Planung GmbH, Elektro A. Haller, Tischlerei Kofler Alois & Co. KG, GR Research GmbH, BIS Berliner Institut für Sozialforschung GmbH, Stiftung St. Elisabeth/Seniorenzentrum im Grieser Hof, Landesverband der Handwerker Südtirol Bozen.

Additionally, the authors would like to thank the consortia of the H2020 Project BERTIM for providing some images in this book. The BERTIM project received funding from the European Union's Horizon 2020 Research and Innovation Programme under Grant Agreement No. 636984.

In addition, some content from the H2020 Project REACH was used. REACH received funding from the European Union's Horizon 2020 Research and Innovation program under Grant Agreement No. 690425.

Furthermore, content from the BMBF Project PASSAge and USA² was used in this book. The project USA² received funding from the German Federal Ministry of Education and Research (BMBF) under Grant No. 16SV6191. The project PASSAge received funding from the German Federal Ministry of Education and Research and VDI/VDE Innovation + Technik GmbH (VDI/VDE-IT).

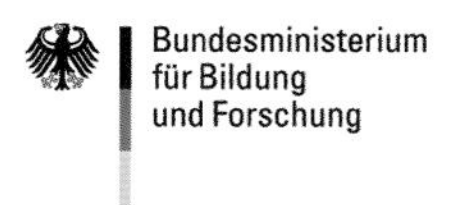

1 Introduction

Aging: no one wants to, but everyone does. Many people are scared of aging mostly because they think of ending up in a bed, doing nothing other than staring at the ceiling and depending on other people who have to sacrifice their free time and strength to care for them. Under these circumstances, not only is the quality of life gone, but also the relationship with relatives can suffer because someone might become a burden.

Scared about this fate, the elderly (and disabled) sometimes wish for suicide or euthanasia. Many need help if their independence is affected because of advanced age. Additionally, euthanasia is illegal in most modern countries.

A new area of research called Ambient (or also Active) Assisted Living (AAL) exists and addresses these concerns. The first ideas in AAL research were introduced in the 1970s, which included technology use from several fields (e.g., robotic solutions). Figure 1.1 shows the first sketches of how such systems could look at that time. Some of these concepts, which were developed and funded by the Japanese Society for the Promotion of Science in 1985, are summarized in [1].

Aging is an unavoidable and natural process. Physicians have investigated whether there is a possibility of slowing down the aging process, but aging is a multifactorial process and cannot easily be manipulated by simple behavioral rules [2]. According to [2], proper nutrition intake, physical activity, and avoidance of obesity and smoking allows for healthy aging and a high quality of life for as long as possible. Antioxidants and caloric restriction promise to positively manipulate the aging process; however, no study has proven any reliable effect. Additionally, there is also a risk of harming the human body by restorative interventions in the aging process, e.g., by caloric restriction [2].

Why do living beings age? According to [2], the aging process is not programmed in the genes of a being, it is more of an evolutionarily successful strategy, which is the outcome of the extrinsic death risk (i.e., the risk of getting killed by accidents or enemies), making it useful to limit the amount of resources for preserving and repairing capabilities.

Sooner or later aging leads to death, and death frees up the bounded biological resources (the different bases, amino acids, proteins, etc.), which supports the development of new life. New life can try to perform better, as explained by Charles Darwin's theory of evolution by natural selection [3]. While physicians and biologists try to find a method that avoids or at least slows down the aging process, engineers work on technological solutions to maintain the independence of the elderly.

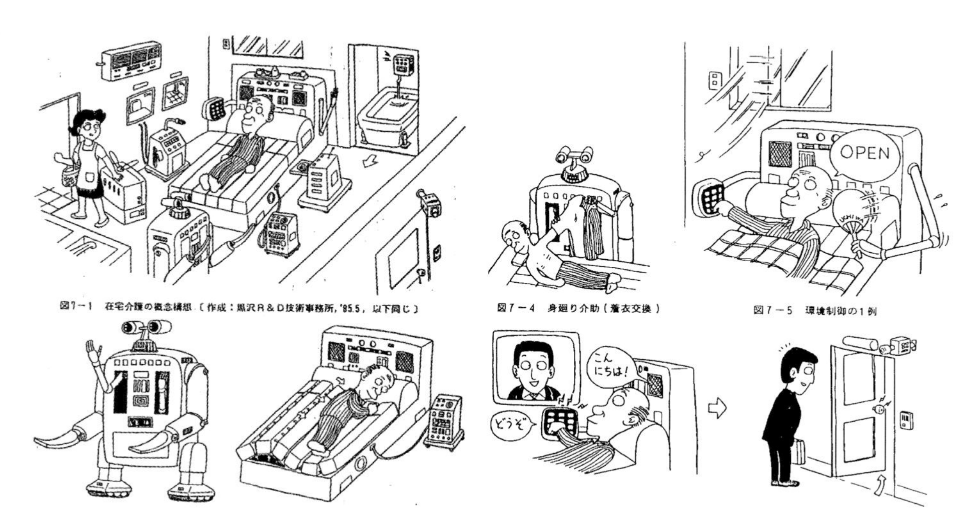

Figure 1.1 The first vision of AAL as developed in Japan 40 years ago[1]. It is a life support system for the elderly. Japan Society for the Promotion of Science. 1985–86.
Source: Thomas Bock

In this volume, current AAL needs and technology are presented to give an outlook on current developments entering the market and research forming the future. This chapter introduces the reader to the background of AAL and its link to robotics.

1.1 Technological Development

This new research field of AAL is therefore a multidisciplinary field connecting researchers from several disciplines (physicians, social researchers, engineers, etc.) to help patients keep their independence. However, aging itself is not the enemy of this research area. Aging leads to multimorbidity [2], which means that the older someone gets, the more fragile the person becomes. Consequently, AAL technology deals with preventing age-related diseases and their secondary diseases or complications (which includes young people) and assisting disabled people, especially regarding age-related diseases. Many wearables and apps have entered the market, mostly using devices like smartphones, which try to support the user in a healthy lifestyle, e.g., apps for weight loss [4], glycosometers, which are add-ons for smartphones [5], etc. Wearables have been used since the first astronauts' flight to space. For example, in space suits during extra-vehicular activities (EVA), according to [6], plethysmographs (for breath detection, as well as lung analysis), Galvanic Skin Resistance (GSR) sensors (for stress detection, e.g., by sweating), skin temperature sensors, and pulse oximeter sensors (for heart rate and oxygen saturation of the blood) were used to check the health status of the astronauts.

However, the technology has now reached a limit, thus allowing researchers to go a step further; instead of just developing new measurement and intervention devices, apartments and buildings can be equipped with sensors and devices that support the user when needed. The apartments and houses become a kind of assistive robot: omnipresent in the environment, but unobtrusively implemented to avoid the feeling of permanent screening. According to [7], researchers working in the AAL field have, in recent years, developed new technological solutions based on ambient intelligence. Ambient intelligence is aiming to empower new capabilities through a digital environment and at the same time being sensitive and adaptive to a user's needs. AAL is not only potentially able to prevent, cure, and improve wellness and health conditions of users, but it also improves safety conditions, e.g., by fall detection, emergency alerts, video surveillance systems, etc. [8]. Also, support in activities of daily living (ADL), e.g., by mobility support and automation, belongs to the field of AAL [9]. Furthermore, communication technology belongs to this field too, as the elderly can connect and communicate more easily with friends and relatives [10]. On the other side, mobile and wearable sensors are more focused on health-related sensor technology, e.g., glucometers, blood pressure devices, and cardiac activities [7]. The idea that robots belong to the field of AAL has already been proven by several research groups, e.g., [11], [12], and [13], aimed to assist movement reduction, fetch objects [14], or transfer support e.g., from bed to wheelchair [15]. According to [7], the smart home is one topic belonging to the AAL sector. Here the analysis and fusion of different types of sensor data helps in obtaining and analyzing information to automate several tasks as well as to increase comfort [16]. Following this approach, modern AAL projects consider not only sensors and devices for automation and comfort, but also the fusing of wearables with smart homes. The entire apartment can be automated, resulting in a robotic apartment. This scenario can be seen as the ultimate fusion of smart homes, wearables, and robotics. More details about such projects are described in Chapter 5.

1.2 Social Development

Why has AAL become so important? The importance of AAL is related to demographic changes, which did not start yesterday. Indeed, the societal demographic changes felt today started at the beginning of the nineteenth century with a growing world population [17].

Technological and (especially) medical knowledge was worse in the nineteenth century than to today. By continued improvements in the medical field, many medications (e.g., arsphenamine [18], and later on penicillin) which allowed for curing deadly diseases, e.g., syphilis [19], have been found. Additionally, when compared to the time before the nineteenth century, child mortality also dramatically changed. For example, the composer Leopold Mozart and his wife Constanze Weber were parents of Maria-Anna Mozart and Wolfgang Amadeus Mozart (see Figure 1.2), as well as of five other children who didn't live beyond 16 years of age. High child mortality was normal. Also, age-related population distribution, as depicted in Figure 1.3, was comparable to a triangle. Families were large and lived together for longer; there was always the possibility that children would take care of their senior parents. Following improved

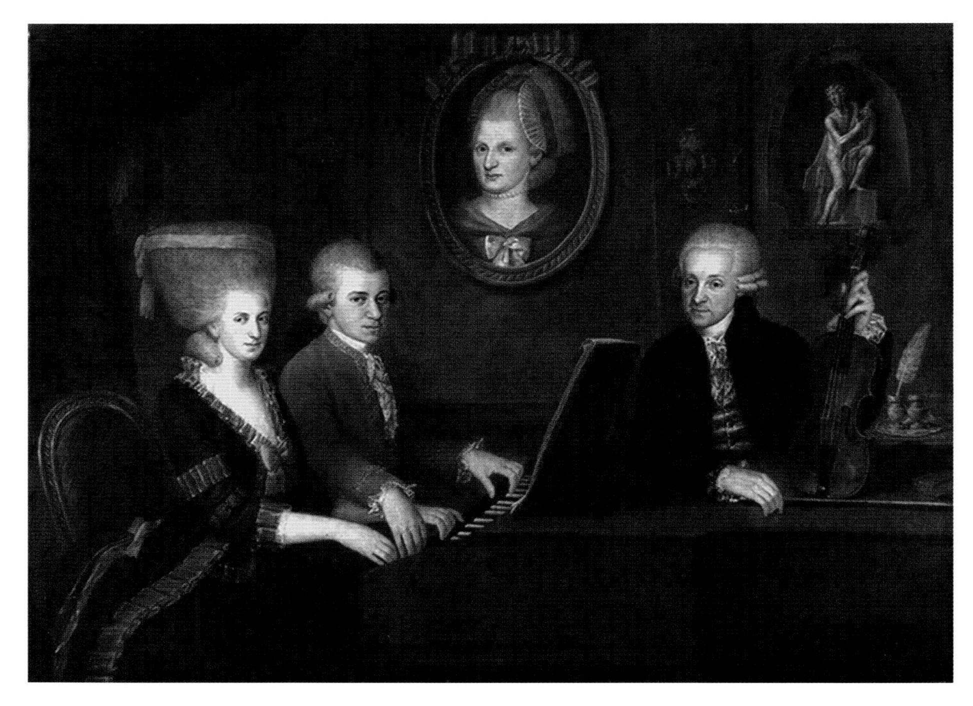

Figure 1.2 Depicted are Leopold Mozart (far right), Wolfgang Amadeus Mozart at the keyboard, next to his sister Maria-Anna Mozart. A portrait of the late mother, Anna Maria, is visible in the center.

Source: Universal History Archive/Getty Images

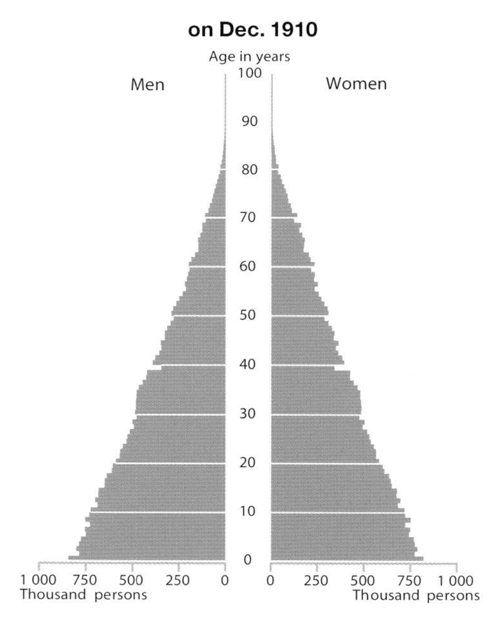

Figure 1.3 Age structure of the population in Germany, December 1910.

Source: Statistisches Bundesamt (Destatis) [20]

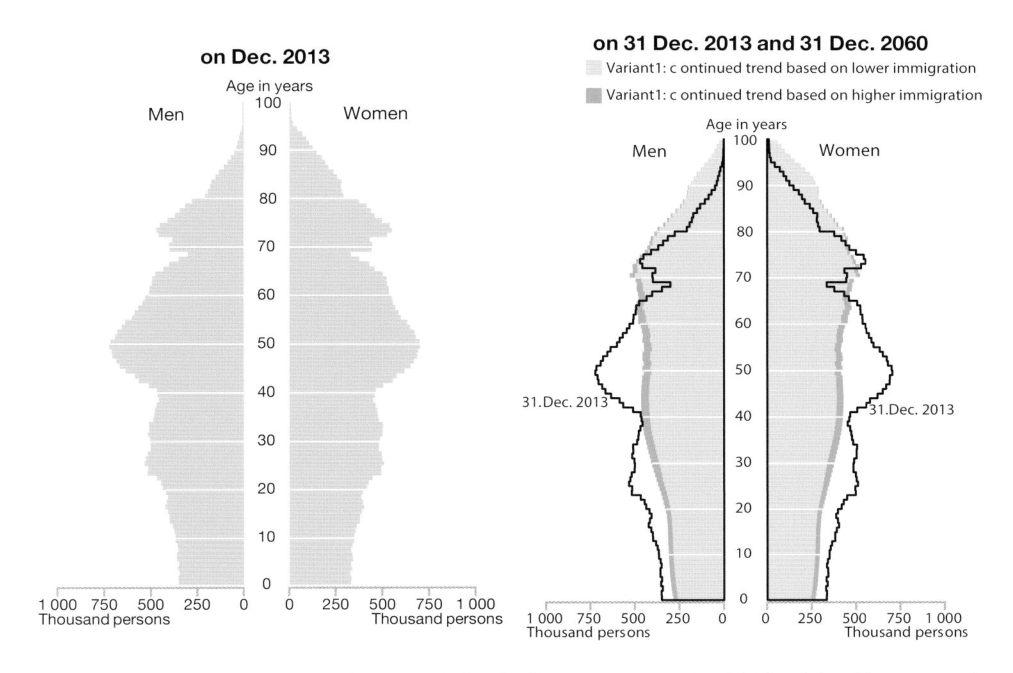

Figure 1.4 Left: Age structure of the population in Germany, December 2013. Right: The expected age structure of the population in Germany, December 2060, compared with 2013.
Source: Statistisches Bundesamt (Destatis) [20]

medication, families started to change because normally children are expensive to take care of. Large families became impoverished because of too many children.

Later on, careers became more important. Parents could earn money and consequently grant one or two children a better life. This led to the fact that children would leave the extended family home and become busy with their own smaller nuclear family. Parents and grandparents normally live in rural areas owing to low living costs, whereas their children move to large cities to work and have better career chances [21]. Therefore, cities like Munich, Hamburg, and Frankfurt [22], become younger, whereas the overall population of industrialized nations is aging.

Figure 1.4 shows the current and future related population distributions. It is clear that the number of young people who can care for the elderly (as compared to Figure 1.3) is extremely reduced, and the situation is projected to worsen.

Caregiver careers are not very highly appreciated by the young population. In Western Europe, poor refugees often work in care homes. However, most care homes now have difficulties in acquiring adequate staff, and the care costs are increasing at the same time. The demographic change is not only a European problem; all industrialized nations are facing the same issue. In Japan and China, the demographic change has an even larger impact. Therefore, many AAL robots and products are already trying to enter the Japanese market (see Section 3.6). To solve the care problem, AAL products have to help elderly patients increase their independence.

1.3 History of Mechatronic/Robotic Environments

It is not surprising that technology is one key to solving the problems caused by demographic change. However, robotics can seem frightening to the elderly, since many do not have a very high affinity for technology. Robots, especially those that resemble humans (also called humanoids) are from a specific point a deterrent for people, especially the elderly [23]. But this perception will change once the next generation needs AAL technology. Additionally, in European stories, robots are normally depicted as evil; e.g., according to [24], movies such as *The Terminator* [25] and *The Animatrix* [26] prove this theory. In Japan, robots have more positive role in literature and film, or at least the "evil" or "bad" roles are more equally distributed between humans and robots [24]. Modern literature and movies, which influence the relationship between people and robots, predict that robots will be accepted in future households. Already some devices prove useful at home, e.g., as vacuum cleaners [27].

In this respect, Japan is more advanced than Europe in two ways: first, Japan is suffering more from demographic change, as already mentioned in Section 1.2, and second, Japan has a very old history in the development of robots, e.g., in form of Karakuri.

According to [28], the first Karakuris was described in the *Konjaku Monogatari* in 1110; it is written that a Karakuri was prepared to supply the farmers in a field (during a drought) with water. Further documents, which prove the early development of robots in the form of Karakuris, can be found in a three-volume book *Karakuri Zui*, written by Hanzō Yorinao in 1796. Compared to the robots later developed in Europe, Karakuri were completely developed out of wood, instead of metal, iron, and screws. Karakuri were also able to express emotion through specialized head movements. Karakuri robots had different abilities, e.g., shooting up to five arrows, when after the fifth arrow the Karakuri express disappointment because of missing the aim (Yumi Karakuri); serving tea (Chahakobi); acrobatics; and stilt walking controlled by a device with rods and strings (Sashigane).

These first robots did not work with electricity or digital processors as those of today. Their technology was strictly mechanical, on the level of developing a clock. Ōno Benkichi (physician and mathematics, 1801–1870) and Tanaka Hisashige (also called Karakuri Giemon, 1799–1881) developed the famous Mannen-Tokei clock. This Japanese clock (see Figure 1.5) adjusted the hours to differing day/night lengths of winter and summer time by asymmetric tooth wheels in the clockwork. The clock adjusted its length mechanically by sliding on the upper half of the clock face or dial six hours before and after noon or midnight. Thus, the mechanics adjusted to the need of the user, which is the same principle applied for the Toyota production system (TPS), which adjusts to need of the worker, and for Japanese cooperative robots since the 1990s. We use a similar approach for our robotic ambience notion described in this volume.

It can be said that all these technologies can adjust to human activity and the environment. In that sense, the Japanese clock system (Figure 1.5) is adapted to the difference of sun light hours in summer and winter.

For example, to control the chahakobi Karakuri robot, which is serving tea, the host and the guest have to define the starting and ending points of the movements together. The Karakuri robots are using potential energy, stored in an updraw coil spring, which

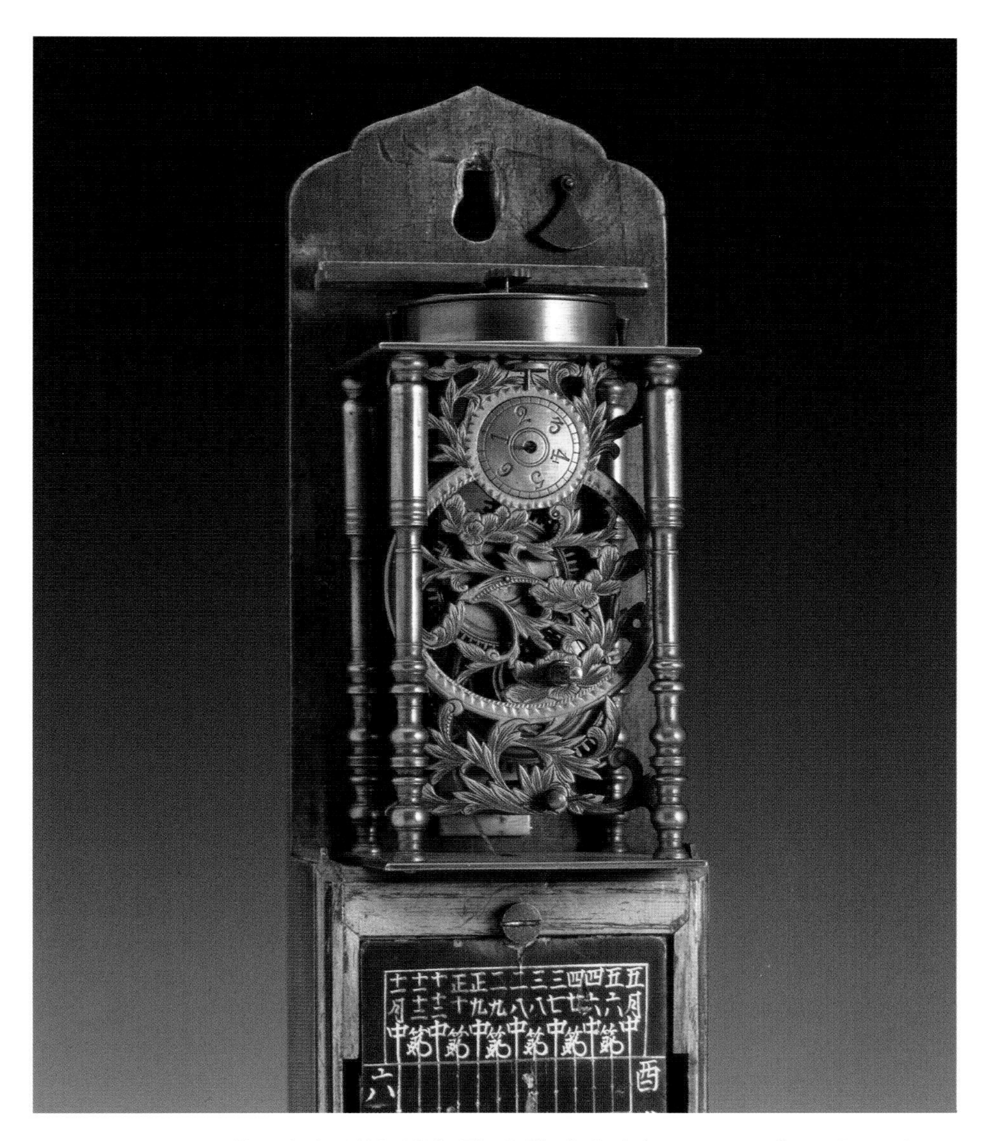

Figure 1.5 Japanese pillar clock, 1800–1870; The "pillar" clock is a type peculiar to Japan, in which the driving weight itself is the time indicator as it falls slowly past a scale of hours mounted below the timekeeping part of the movement. The hour numerals are adjustable by hand to allow for the varying hours of the day and night through the year. The Japanese system of "temporal hours" timekeeping until 1870 divided the day and night each into six equal "hours." The length of these "hours" differed throughout the year as the seasons changed.
Source: SSPL/Getty Images

will be transformed into kinetic energy. Additionally, the feet of the robot pretend to walk. The complex mechanism is triggered by a plate in the hands of the chahakobi Karakuri robot, where the teacup is placed. These very first pressure sensors enabled the users to trigger when the robot shall move 180° around and go back.

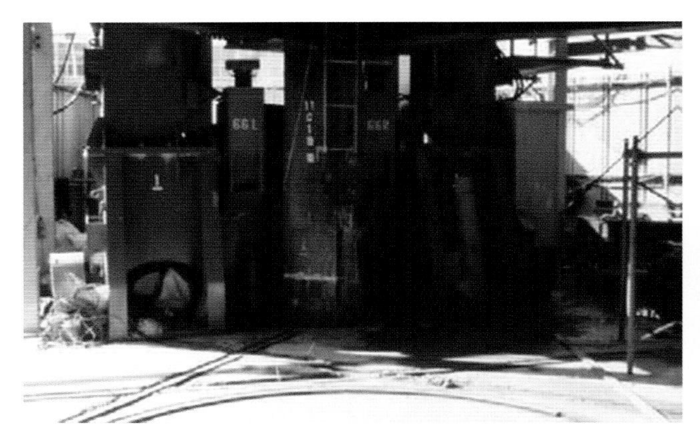
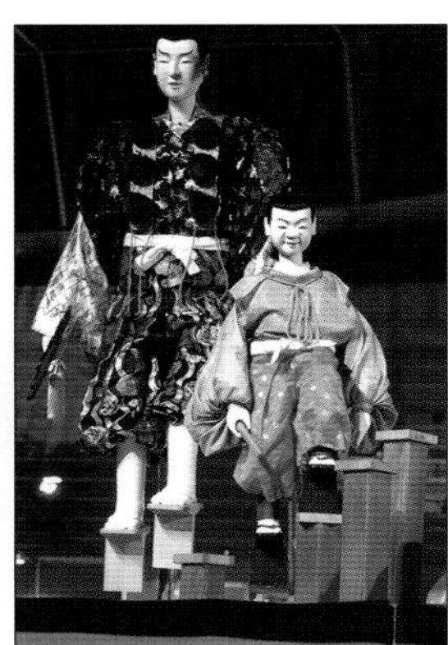

Figure 1.6 Left: Sashigane lifting press.
Source: Prof. Bock
Right: Karasu Tengu-mechanical puppet.
Source: Kurita KAKU/Gamma-Rapho via Getty Images

Therefore, Karakuri robots include the user (or guest) in their show and put the guest at the center of the attention, which can (and should) easily laugh by the mistakes of the Karakuri robot. The life expectancy of the Karakuri is between 50 and 100 years, and their modular construction allows for easy repair by disassembling. All these aspects have the psychological success that in Japan robots are not a threat to the population. Therefore, the Japanese philosophy of Kaizen (which means continuous improvement) fused with the Karakuri create the philosophy of Karakuri-Kaizen, the basis for a sustainable and a highly efficient production process in modern factories of Japan.

This functional principal of Karakuri is especially visible in construction areas. On high-rise construction sites, the devices used are very similar to the Karakuri principal; their rotation, lifting, and rope mechanisms are partly automated. The only difference here is that these devices are digitally controlled.

At the end of the 1970s, the Shimizu Company started to experiment with construction robots. Computer-controlled CNC processes for Japanese timber engineering has existed since the 1960s. The Sashigane control from the Karakuri, which has been available since the 1700s in Kabuki Theatre (during the Edo period), is the basis for the Sakauchi method used in Japan (see Figure 1.6).

The Karakuri principle is also found in buildings in different occurrences, e.g., the Zashiki Karakuri, a small device for the reception room (mostly only for private use), or the Yashiki Karakuri or Ninja Yashiki, where the whole house is equipped with manipulability mechanisms (Figure 1.10). Therefore, in houses from the Mochizuki Izumonokami, in Kōka at Kyōto, from 1487, different specialties like hidden subfloors, folding ladders, double walls, etc., are implemented. Most famous are the rotating walls (donden gaeshi), which are access points to hidden rooms and floors, or cavities to hide weapons (yukashita mono kakushi), flush doors (kakushido), etc. This approach could be named Karakuri-Architecture, Apartment-Karakuri, or Building-Karakuri,

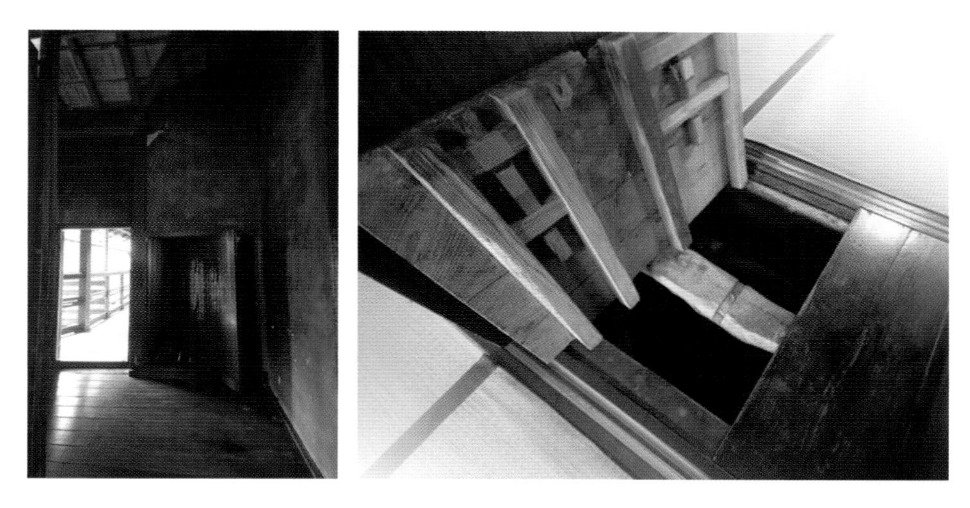

Figure 1.7 Pictures from the Kouka-ninjya house in Kōka showing a revolving wall (left) and a trap (right) for hiding from possible enemies.

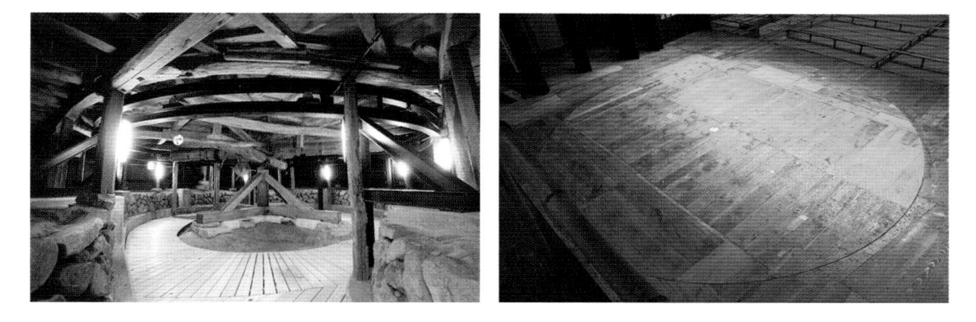

Figure 1.8 Revolving stage or Mawari-butai Karakuri.
Images from Izushi Eraikukan[30]

which means to unobtrusively embed different mechanisms into the environment, a similar approach to the AAL technology of the future (more details can be found in Section 2.2). A good example of the integration of devices is the Kouka-ninjya house in Kōka [29], which was a former inn for feudal lords or ninjas. Here, many "secret" devices for hiding can be found if the situation required an escape (see Figure 1.7).

The Karakuri technology has also influenced Europe, e.g., use of the rotating stage in theater during the Edo epoch (1602–1868) was used in the Kabuki Theater play "Nakamura Denshichi." Furthermore, the prototype of the modern rotating stage has been used by Namiki Shoza (1730–1773) in the theater play "Sanjikoku Yofune no hajimari" at the Za-Kabuik-Theater in Ōsaka in 1758. The rotating stage, which found its perfection in 1848, had two opposite rotating stages, and was introduced in Europe at the end of the nineteenth century. By using the Karakuri mechanism, whole stage sets can arise in seconds, which allows the whole stage to work as a Karakuri mechanism, proving once more the success of unobtrusive implementation of complex technology into the environment. The invention was named as "mawari-butai" (see Figure 1.8) and there are still some that are performing as the Eirakukan in Izushi [30]. Even today this is inspiring latest research projects, which try to develop robotic rooms by

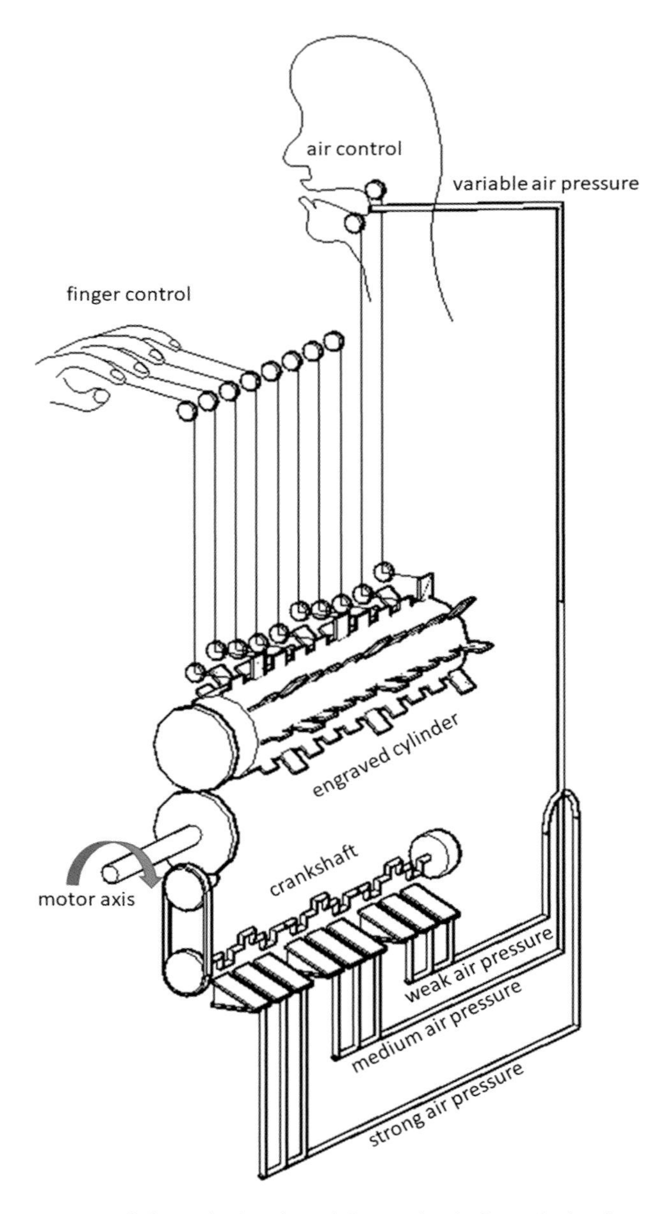

Figure 1.9 Schematic drawing of the mechanic flute-playing invented by Vacaunson.
Source: Kepa Iturralde

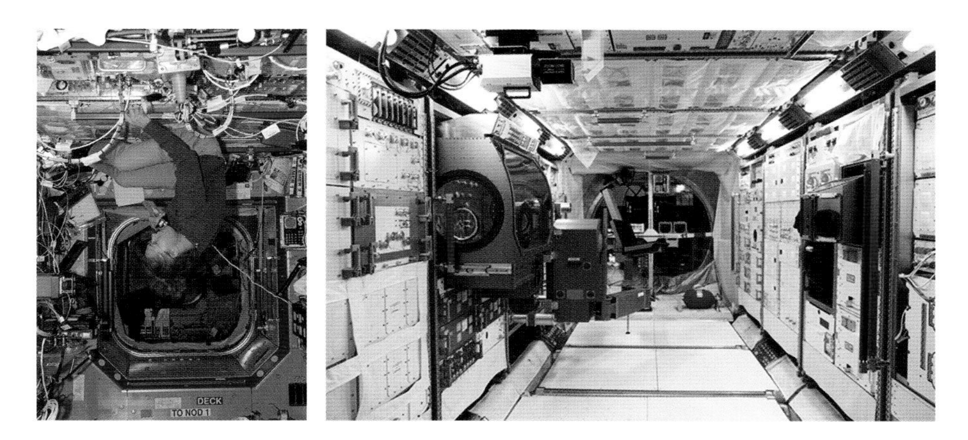

Figure 1.10 Left: NASA astronaut Sandy Magnus works in the US lab or Destiny addition of the International Space Station.
Source: NASA via Getty Images
Right: General view of the Columbus simulator in the ESA Planetary Robotics Lab.
Source: Dean Mouhtaropoulos/Getty Images

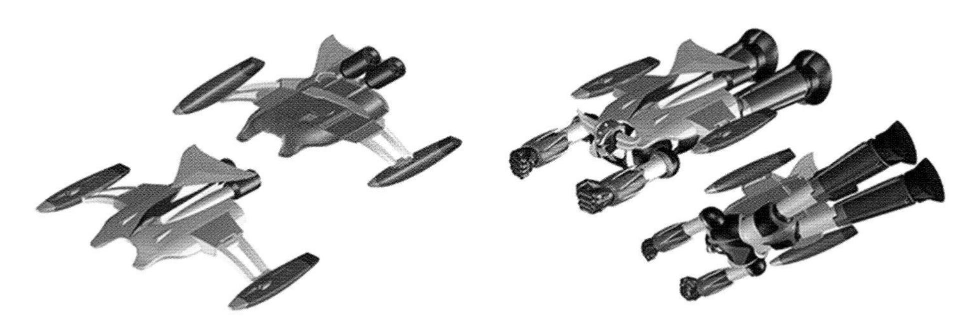

Figure 1.11 Bandai´s transformers recall the ancient Karakuri concept.
Courtesy of Bandai and Dynamic Planning, Toei Animation ©

implementing high tech robotic devices and sensors unobtrusively into the environment [31] (see also Chapter 5).

In Europe, the modern history of automats probably starts with Jacques de Vacaunson when he invented a mechanic flute-playing device that blew air through a real flute (see Figure 1.9) [32] [33].

The modern crewed spacecraft (Figure 1.10) can be considered a modern version of the Nijo Jinya building [29], where mechanical devices are integrated on the interior living environment. The astronauts can operate with these machines and devices for everyday living and to accomplish their work.

Finally, we can find the new modern version of the Karakuri concept in the transformer toys developed and commercialized by the Japanese company Bandai [34].

2 Basic Knowledge, Strategies, and Procedures

In this chapter, we present a background on the state of the art regarding Ambient/Active Assisted Living (AAL) related topics (i.e., Ambient Sensing, Medical Technology, and Geriatrics and Sociology). Later in the book we present the basis for current, new, and common technologies on the market (presented in Chapter 4), and ongoing research in AAL (examples presented in Chapter 5). The presented interdisciplinary content consists of social, engineering, medical, electrical, and mechatronics science, and together, they encompass the field of AAL, as well as eHealth.

In recent years, AAL and eHealth have become important topics because of increased life expectancy. Even though this topic is age related, young people have already started to have a high interest in this field due to the potential for the prevention of age-related diseases.

Therefore, this chapter introduces the technological feasibility for Ambient Sensing and will be linked with the possibilities of medical technology and the necessary geriatrics background. At the end, the potential of technology of robotics in this field is presented.

2.1 Basic Knowledge in the Field of Ambient Sensing

When people enter a stage of physical and cognitive decline, typically associated with the natural aging process, the independent exercise of Activities of Daily Living (ADLs) becomes increasingly difficult [35]. If sensing and intervention technologies are not developed, this decline may progress prematurely and unnecessarily to the point when affected groups will eventually not live independently at home and become a burden on family members and institutionalized nursing-care systems. These considerations are particularly important since every emerging industrial nation is experiencing demographic change problems [36]. In this aspect, Ambient Sensing solutions could undoubtedly contribute to addressing these emerging problems.

Ambient Sensing refers to environments populated with sensors responsive and sensitive to the presence of people. An environment populated with electronic elements and microsystems can undoubtedly contribute to enhancing the independence of the elderly by introducing a degree of ambient assistance. Monitoring people's movements in complex environments, analyzing the resulting motion patterns, and understanding people's gestures corresponds to a high level of visual competence that can most appropriately be identified as Ambient Intelligence (AmI) [37]. Thus, Ambient Sensing – belonging to the AmI research umbrella – builds upon advances in sensors and sensor networks, pervasive computing, and artificial intelligence. Because these contributing fields have experienced tremendous growth in the last few years, Ambient Sensing has strengthened and expanded, revolutionizing daily human life by making people's surroundings flexible and adaptive. Technologies are deployed to make computers disappear in the background, while the human moves into the foreground in complete control of the augmented environment. Ambient Sensing systems are a user-centric paradigm, supporting a variety of artificial intelligence methods and works pervasively, nonintrusively, and transparently to aid the user. They support and promote interdisciplinary research encompassing the technological, scientific, and artistic fields, thus creating a virtual support for embedded and distributed intelligence. They will eventually become invisible, embedded in our natural surroundings, present whenever we need them, enabled by simple and effortless interactions, attuned to all our senses, adaptive to users, context-sensitive, and autonomous.

The basic idea consists of a distributed layered architecture enabling omnipresent communication, and an advanced human–machine communication protocol. The Ambient Sensing paradigm sets the principles to design a pervasive and transparent infrastructure capable of observing people without interfering with their lives but at the same time adapting to the needs of the user. It must be noted that populating a home environment with sensors must be performed following a space-efficient utilization scheme. Elderly people, and especially the ones using assistive devices such as wheelchairs and rollators, require increased barrier-free space for mobility purposes.

In the following sections, an overview about the rule of vision systems as well as radio-frequency identification (RFID) technology in this context is provided in order to explain the different underlying technologies used in the realization of such systems, and their corresponding application areas.

2.1.1 Vision Systems

Vision is arguably the strongest of the senses in humans and in many other creatures. It allows us to fully understand the surrounding environment by providing spatial information of objects around us. With this amazing ability, we can determine the position, identity, and status of the various objects in the environment, so that we can interact with and react to various unexpected events. It is therefore reasonable that we attempt to give a sense of vision to the machines in order to turn them into even more useful and efficient tools. Many vision-based sensors have therefore been developed throughout the years. Three-dimensional (3D) vision systems base their operation on the collection of stereoscopic image pairs and on decoding the depth of information by examining the relative displacements of objects within a pair of images, relative to each other. This process is called stereo-photogrammetry. The observation, using our eyes, allows us to perceive the relative distance (depth) of objects that enter our field of vision. However, the human brain is the mechanism that is responsible for successfully decoding the depth information, i.e., the stereoscopic image pair, giving us the ability of depth perception. Conversely, in stereoscopic vision systems, an algorithm that can analyze the digital images taken by a stereo camera pair and recover the important depth information by sampling the areas which are illustrated in the optical scene must be devised. Depth estimation in a scene using image pairs acquired by a stereo camera setup is one of the important tasks of stereo vision systems.

Disparity map extraction of an image is a computationally demanding task; practical real-time hardware-based algorithms require high device utilization recourse usage, and depending on their disparity level operational ranges, this may lead to significant power consumption. Apart from digital camera sensors, other technologies which base their "visual" sensing performance on laser, such as Light Detection and Ranging (LiDAR), or infrared such as Depth Sensors have also been developed.

2.1.2 RFID Technology

In recent years, RFID technology has moved from insignificant into conventional applications that aid in simplifying the handling of items and objects. RFID enables identification from a distance, and unlike the earlier barcodes technology, it functions without requiring a line of sight or a specific visual pattern to be detected, recorded, and processed [38]. RFID tags (see Figure 2.1) support a larger set of unique IDs than barcodes and can incorporate additional data such as manufacturer, product type, and even measure environmental factors such as temperature. Furthermore, RFID systems can discern many different tags located in the same general area without human assistance. In contrast, consider a supermarket checkout counter, where the personnel must orient each barcoded item toward a laser scanner reader in order to identify it. If all items had an RFID tag attached on them, the checkout process on the counter could have been fully automated without explicitly requiring human assistance.

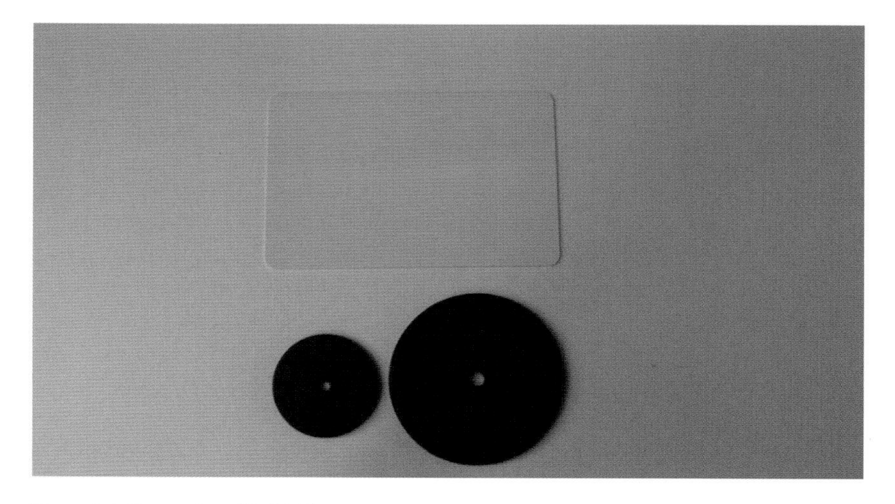

Figure 2.1 Exemplary RFID Tag.

Many types of RFIDs exist, but at the highest level we can divide RFID devices into two broad classes [39]: active and passive tags. Active tags require a power source, i.e., they are either connected to a powered infrastructure or use energy stored in an integrated battery. One example of an active tag is the transponder attached to an aircraft that identifies its national origin. However, batteries make the cost, size, and lifetime of active tags impractical for most small-scale applications. Passive RFID tags are thus preferred because they don't require an external supply source. The tags also have huge operational lifetimes and are tiny enough to fit into a practical, adhesive label.

A passive tag consists of three parts: an antenna, a processing unit attached to the antenna, and some form of encapsulation. A tag reader is responsible for powering and communicating with a tag, which is attached either to a personal computer or to a digital communication network. The tag antenna captures energy and transfers the tag's ID. The tag's processing unit is responsible for coordinating the communication and transmission process. The encapsulation maintains the tag integrity and protects the antenna and processing unit from environmental conditions or damage.

In a home environment, this technology can be utilized to assist elderly people by providing them with a real-time inventory of their high priority items. Experiments conducted during the proposed study, revealed the efficiency of this "invisible" technology, and the variety of potential applications to which this technology can contribute. By combining computerized databases and inventory controls linked through digital communication networks spread across the home environment and across a global set of locations, RFID technology can efficiently pinpoint individual items as they move between locations, warehouses, vehicles, and stores.

2.2 Basic Knowledge in the Field of Medical Technology

Life quality and health are very closely related to each other. It does not matter how rich or poor someone is, as soon as their health is gone, they suffer. Therapy is necessary to successfully cure a person. The type of therapy is dependent on the disease, and therefore it is a major task for a physician to identify the cause of a disease and then decide together with the patient how to recover or at least treat the disease.

Depending on the kind and stage of a disease, it may happen that the affected becomes unconscious or comatose suddenly and without any warning symptoms. This happens with diseases that have silent symptoms and break out suddenly. For example, heart attacks can be a result of a permanently high blood pressure. To treat a person, the cause of the disease must first be identified. An anamnesis (if possible) in combination with first measurements (e.g., blood pressure, pulse, glucose, and ECG) allow the physician to find the proper treatment, and sometimes to identify additional health risks. For example, type II diabetes is a typical disease, which normally in a physical examination gets accidentally diagnosed [40] by a physician because of other reasons. However, this means regular physical examinations increase the chances to recognize the beginning of a disease at an early stage, where the chances of a cure are high. The field of medical technology therefore focuses a lot on identifying diseases.

More people, old and young, are aware of these facts. Therefore, wearables, which measure physiological parameters, have successfully entered the consumer market. Wearables, however, tend to be forgotten to wear, and many people feel that wearing them all day is inconvenient. In order to improve health screening and to increase the security of the user, a new strategy has started in this field of research: the unobtrusive implementation of health sensors in the environment.

Sensors must be noninvasive for both physicians and patients and designed to work in the background when implementing health sensors into the user environment. In the following sections, devices used for noninvasive diagnostics are introduced, which are highly interesting because they can be unobtrusively implemented into the user's environment. The possibilities are too large to present every type of measurement; however, we will give an overview of the most important measurements with regards to AAL and eHealth.

2.2.1 Pulse Oximetry

Pulse oximetry is used to measure pulse and oxygen saturation at the same time. To do this, a sensor has to be attached on the earlobe or finger [41], or at the heel for newborn and premature babies. The sensor consists of a light sensor and an emitting source. There are two possibilities of how the sensor measures and receives pulse and oxygen blood saturation data: either by the transmission of the tissue from the emitted light, or by remission (see Figure 2.2).

The pulse is then counted by the arrival of the absorbed light on the photodiode. The emitted light gets absorbed by a blood wave, which is passing by the measurement spot.

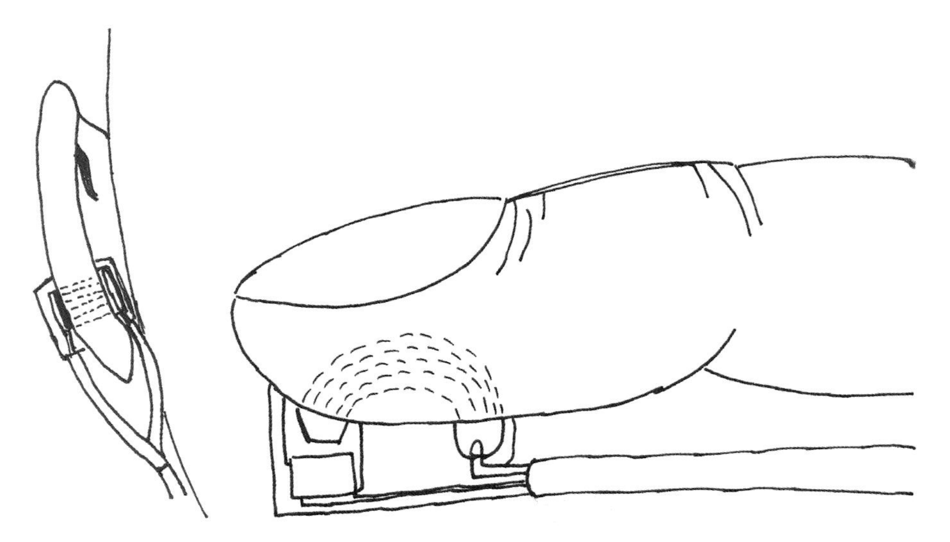

Figure 2.2 Left: Exemplary sketch of pulse oximetry on the earlobe with light transmission. Right: Exemplary sketch of pulse oximetry on the finger with light remission.
Source: J. Güttler

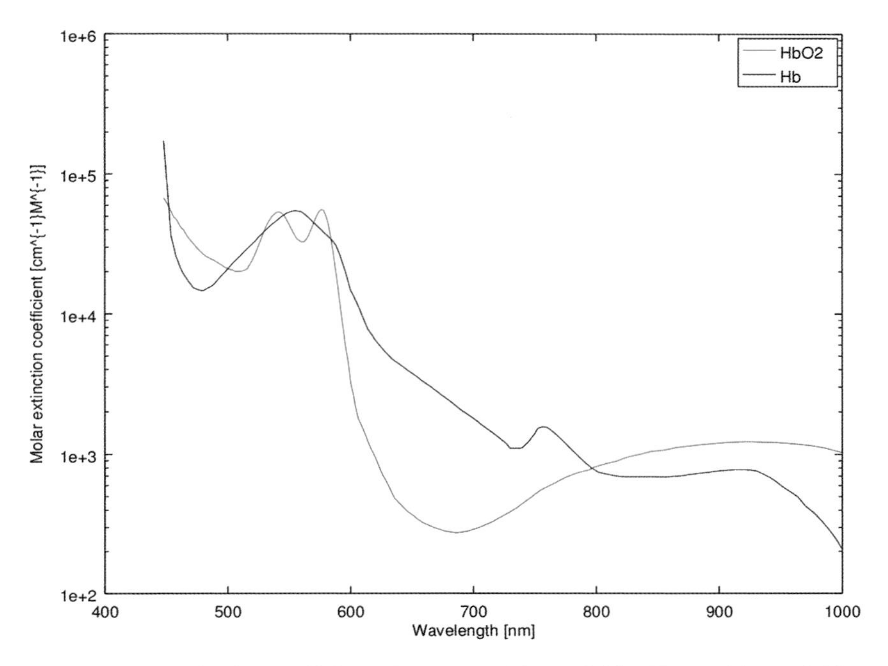

Figure 2.3 The extinction coefficient of unsaturated hemoglobin (Hb), and hemoglobin saturated with oxygen (HbO_2).
Source: Adapted from S. Prahl, "Tabulated Molar Extinction Coefficient for Haemoglobin in Water," Oregon Medical Laser Center, No. 4, 1998

Usually for this technology, an LED-emitting light to a photodiode is used [42]. To make the signal usable, a power amplifier is normally used for an analog low-pass filter, which amplifies the signal [43].

To measure the oxygen saturation of the blood, two LEDs are necessary: one should emit light at 660 nm (red light), and the other LED at 950 nm (infrared). The reason for this is due to the extinction coefficient of blood (shown in Figure 2.3, data source [44]). When saturated with oxygen, the erythrocytes absorb more infrared light and absorb less light at 660 nm. The 950 nm LED is used to get a relative value for the reference measurement Hb, whereas 660 nm is used for the HbO_2. Using Eq. (2.1) allows for calculating the precentral saturation in relation to the overall hemoglobin.

$$SaO_2 = \frac{HbO_2}{Hb + HbO_2} \cdot 100\% \tag{2.1}$$

However, this sensor has two weak points; heavy movements can easily disturb the measurement and, at the end, the device can only detect how much of the blood is saturated. Normally the oxygen is binding with the hemoglobin, which the erythrocytes carry. However, other gases like carbon dioxide bind much more strongly than oxygen to the blood. This leads to a perfect measurement result, although the blood does not carry oxygen. This dangerous life situation, which, for example, can occur in response to a fire gas intoxication, cannot be detected using this technology.

Also, smoking can lead to wrong results. A person who smokes during a measurement period will have 100 percent saturation. However, the true saturation will be visible after some time and will drop to around 95 percent. In [41], the following thresholds for pulse oximetry are defined: A healthy person normally has 95–100 percent saturation. People who have 94 percent saturation or lower normally suffer from hypoxia and need treatment. People with a saturation of less than 90 percent are a medical emergency case.

2.2.2 Blood Pressure Meter

Those who have used a blood pressure meter know that the device gives three values: the systolic blood pressure, the diastolic blood pressure, and the pulse. In the past, physicians and caretakers measured the blood pressure by palpation (according to the Riva–Rocci method) with a cuff. Therefore, e.g., the caretaker, or physician, must find the pulse, e.g., on the wrist of the patient. Once the pulse has been found, the cuff, placed on the upper arm, gets pumped (using a small hand pump) until the pressure is large enough to close the brachial artery [45]. This stops the blood flow to the hand, which is not very convenient if the pressure is high for too long.

Of course, now there is no noticeable pulse. Slowly opening the valve on the cuff leads to a slow reduction of the pressure, which the cuff uses to close the artery. The nurse, or physician, has to wait until the first pulse wave is noticeable on the wrist: this is the blood pressure that is strong enough to open the artery for a very short moment. This value is called the systolic blood pressure. This value is the highest pressure and marks the pressure occurring during a heart contraction.

However, there is also a constant low blood pressure while the heart is not contracting. This value is known as the diastolic blood pressure. To also measure the diastolic value, physicians and caretakers use a stethoscope to hear the Korotkoff-sound (auscultatory measurement).

These Korotkoff-sounds, which sound similar to a heartbeat but are of distinct origins, are the result of turbulences, which occur when the cuff is narrowing the artery (see Figure 2.4) [46]. As soon as the vessel is able to send blood through the occlusion (caused by the pumped cuff), this sound occurs and marks the systolic value (as it is with the palpatory measurement). The Korotkoff-sound stops as soon as the turbulence stops and the blood continues with a laminar flow, which is achieved as soon as the pressure of the cuff is weaker than the lower blood pressure (the diastolic value). This means that the last Korotkoff-sound the physician or caretaker hears, while reducing the cuff pressure by the valve, marks the diastolic blood pressure.

However, both methods (palpation and auscultation) are very subjective measurement methods dependent on the sensibility and hearing abilities of the person taking the measurement. Herein, this measurement method has been automated. The device in principle consists of an automated pump and a pressure sensor (e.g., a capacitive pressure sensor) measures the pulse. The device pumps the cuff to close the artery and then stepwise reduces the pressure (as depicted in Figure 2.5). Once the cuff has a larger pressure than the cuff, the pulse oscillation increases, which the blood pressure

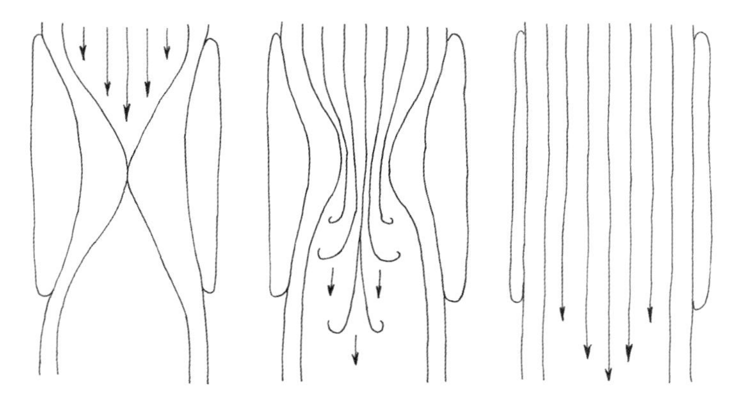

Figure 2.4 Left: No blood flow, because the cuff pressure is higher than the systolic blood pressure. Center: Turbulence blood flow, which causes the Korotkoff-sounds, because the cuff pressure is between systolic and diastolic blood pressure. Right: Laminar blood flow, because the cuff pressure is lower than the diastolic blood pressure.
Source: J. Güttler

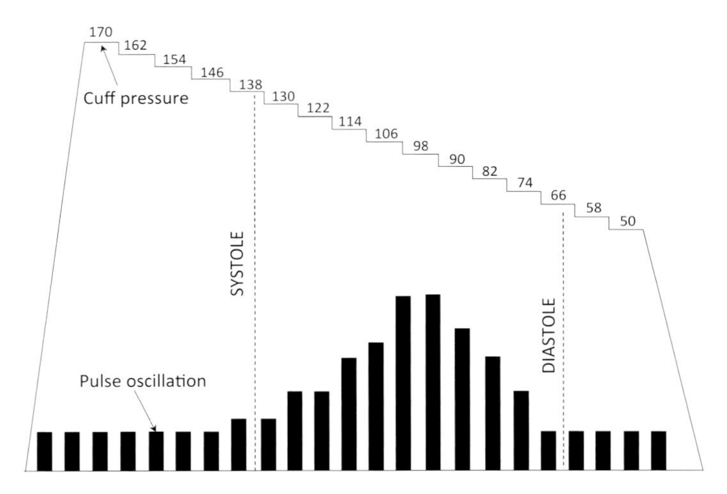

Figure 2.5 Exemplary sketch describing the working principle of a blood pressure meter.
Source: J. Güttler

meter marks as a systolic value. Once the oscillation strength returns to its normal level, the device marks the cuff pressure as a diastolic value.

However, the most precise method to measure a blood pressure is the invasive blood pressure measurement. Here, the pressure sensor is not attached to a cuff; it is directly attached via a catheter or cannula to the arterial blood. Using this method allows care staff or a physician to differentiate the blood pressure in the region and system. The blood pressure meters, as described in this section, measures the high-pressure system. However, the blood pressure of the veins belonging to the low blood pressure system is not measured by the commercial devices [47].

Normally the blood pressure should give a result of 100 mmHg up to 140 mmHg (optimal 120 mmHg) for the systolic, and less than 100 mmHg for the diastolic blood pressure value. However, the blood pressure is also dependent on the body region, as well as of the kind of blood pressure system.

2.2.3 Temperature Measurement

The body temperature is a physiological parameter, which can change according to the environment or the health condition. An increased temperature, caused by diseases like influenza, is called a fever. Often, a fever is part of the defensive response of the immune system, with the objective to kill intruding microbiological organisms like bacteria or viruses [48]. Although this means that a fever is supporting the curing process, a fever can be dangerous if the temperature is above 43°C [49]. Therefore, a fever is a good measure of someone's health. For the elderly, it is specifically important since high fever can harm the cardiovascular circulation, and this often needs to be suppressed.

To identify a fever, touching the forehead may be enough. However, this can be a very imprecise method. Fortunately, fever measurement devices are very cheap, and nearly every drugstore sells such devices. Mercury-in-glass thermometers (see Figure 2.6), which measure the temperature related expansion of the liquid, have now been replaced by the most common digital version (see Figure 2.6) of this measurement device (which measures by a thermistor). The disadvantage of these devices is the fact that they need up to 5 minutes to receive a result. Measurement areas are axillar, oral, and rectal, whereas axillar is not considered to be the most precise measurements area [50], but the axillar measurement is one of the most convenient measurement areas. Of course, there are also other measurement areas, which are quite inconvenient or even painful, e.g., rectal [51].

However, user impatience (especially in small children) often leads to false measurement results. Therefore, devices which measure the fever very fast and reliably by

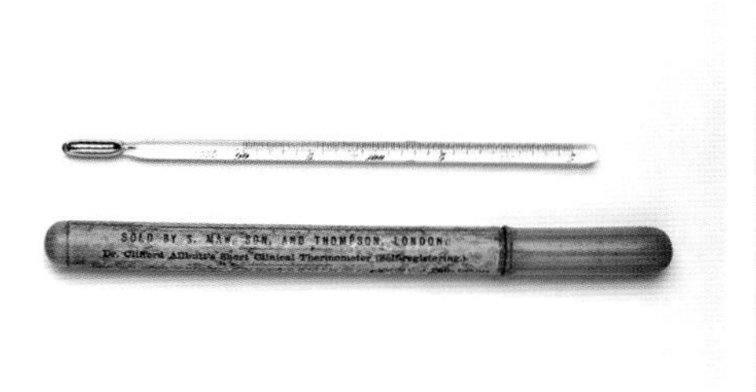

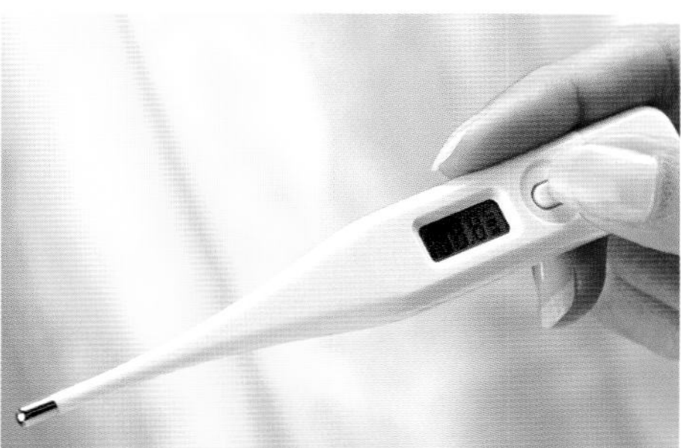

Figure 2.6 Left: mercury-in-glass thermometer.
Source: SSPL/Getty Images
Right: digital thermometer.
Source: BSIP/UIG via Getty Images

infrared on the eardrum ([52], [53], [54]) now exist. However, there is a high risk with this device related to wrong measurements, e.g., by wrongly holding the tympanic fever measurement device, which is then measuring the meatus, instead of the ear drum. An additional disadvantage is that all the mentioned body temperature measurement methods or devices need direct body contact, which leads to hygiene problems. For example, [55] points out the importance of sterilizing these devices, if they are to be used for more than one person.

Therefore, thermometers which measure fever on the forehead without direct contact by infrared also exist. Depending on the environmental temperature, the accuracy of this kind of measurement may be compromised [56], [57]. On the other side, these kinds of devices allow a fast and hygienic measurement of the body temperature. In the last years, this aspect of fast and hygienic measurements became very important not just for the health care, eHealth, and AAL sectors, but also with regards to travel of tourists and business people through different climatic areas. Traveling brings together people of different immune system strengths, which in return supports the development of epidemics and pandemics (e.g., the influenza pandemic in 2009 [58]). Since influenza is a health and even life risk for the elderly [59], thermal cameras have been used at airports for quick mass screening [60]. Therefore, it is not surprising that there are several studies (e.g., [61], [62], [63]), which have investigated the usage and reliability of thermal cameras for fever measurement.

2.2.4 Glucometers and Their Measurement Possibilities

Type II diabetes is the most common metabolic disease in the world, which can lead to blindness and limb loss [64]. Therefore, Glucometers have become important devices in a lot of homes. The general measurement principle is normally based on enzymes, which react only with the sugar molecules in the blood.

According to [65], the enzymes are immobilized on a platinum electrode, which must get in contact with the blood. The enzymes will then react (oxidize) with the glucose and release electrons. The glucometer finally measures the current when the freed electrons pass the device to equalize the potential difference of the electrodes. The current is proportional to the glucose concentration in the blood.

The enzymes and the electrodes are one-way products, and mostly sold as strips, which get connected by plug and play into the glucose meter (see Figure 2.7). The analysis is normally done by the glucometer itself. To get out the blood drop, the user must pierce the skin to get blood out of the capillaries (i.e., minimal invasive measurement). As the end user normally prefers to centralize functions in one device (instead of having several measurements at home), add-ons which use the smartphone to display the result exist.

However, although this method is reliable in measuring the blood sugar level (very important especially for people who are consuming insulin), this method is very inconvenient. Alternative measurement methods have been investigated. A new product to receive the same results is the glucose scanner, which must be held next to a patch. The patch itself consists of a very small needle and a small circuit, which measures and

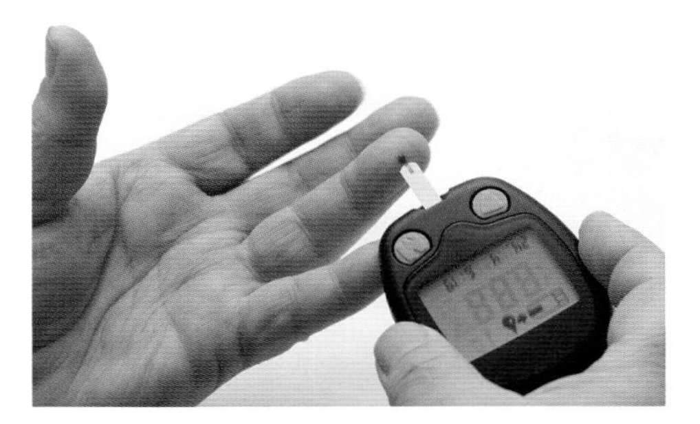

Figure 2.7 A glucose meter, including the test stripe, where the blood drop must be inserted. Source: Eldemir/Getty Images

transmits the results as soon as the scanner is close enough. The patches must be replaced only once every two weeks, thus reducing injury to the skin.

However, as diabetes starts mostly silent (i.e., without clinical symptoms [40]), there is an interest to measure just for prevention. With diabetes, there is no big alternative to pricking the skin daily, but for people who just want to prevent diabetes, this is unacceptable. An alternative to checking blood sugar is checking sugar levels in urine. If the sugar concentration in the blood exceeds the renal threshold of ~180 mg/dl, glucose will be excreted in the urine. Normally a urine test stripe can prove glucose exists in the urine by an enzyme reaction, which changes the color accordingly.

In Japan, toilets are equipped with the glucometers to measure the glucose in the toilets (see Section 4.3).

2.2.5 Electrical Biosignals

Up-to-date electoral biosignals are one of the most important, non-invasive measurements methods. The electrocardiogram (ECG) is probably the most used; many are used in hospitals as well as in emergency departments. The ECG measures the sum of the electrical potential of all heart cells. The measurement of the Einthoven triangle was defined by Einthoven in 1913 [66]. The signal is measured on the hands and on the left feet, as shown in Figure 2.8.

Since the generated signal is very weak, a differential amplifier linking two electrodes with each other is used. The measurement vector then determines the amplitude, and the more parallel it is to the electrical heart vector, the higher the amplitude is (see Figure 2.9).

Three measurements to investigate the current activity are possible with these three leads. Following the definition of Goldberger, the augmented voltage leads aVR, aVL, and aVF (see Figure 2.10), which allow a more detailed investigation, have been introduced. Of course, there are more possibilities to investigate the heart using only ECG by appropriated electrode placing (e.g., according to Wilson, Caprera circle [67], and Nehb [68]). The ECG has already entered the private eHealth market via several

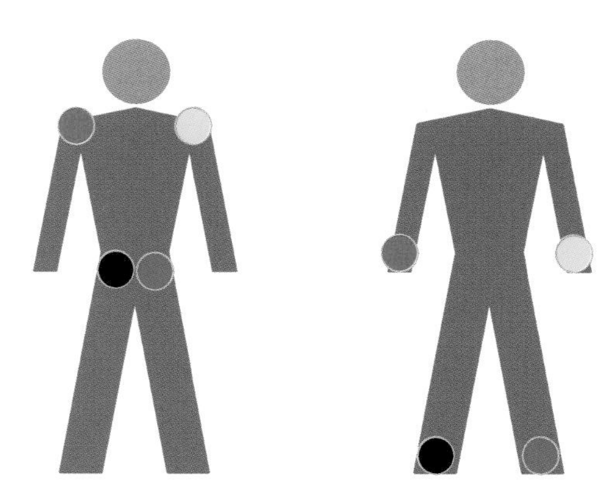

Figure 2.8 Possible electrode placement areas for Einthoven and Goldberger lead measurements.

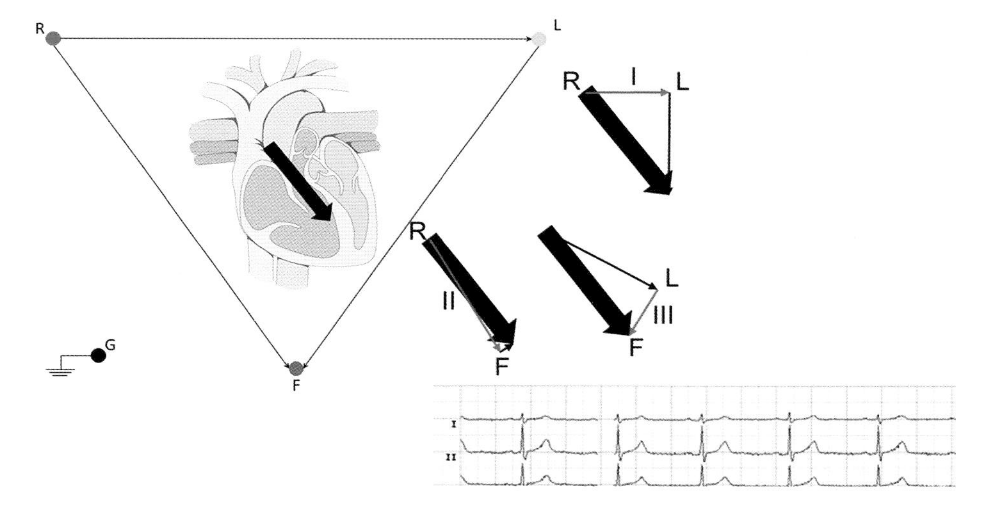

Figure 2.9 The electrical heart vector (black arrow) and its vectorial relation of the Einthoven I, II, and III leads, which ultimately influences the ECG amplitude.

devices like jogging watches, where the pulse button and the watch back are electrodes, or in training devices like ergometers (e.g., embedded in the handlebars).

The difference between the ECG and the electromyogram (EMG) is in the embedded filters. The EMG is normally much stronger in the signal of the ECG and normally filtered. EMG works the same as the ECG but focuses on detecting the electrical signal of the muscles. The EMG is an important sensing device in the medical area and also in the future of eHealth and AAL. For example, the first implementation can be found in exoskeletons, which serves, for example, as orthosis [69] [70].

The Electrooculography (EOG) and the Electroencephalography (EEG) are mainly used for investigating sleeping behavior (e.g., the EOG is used to identify the rapid eye

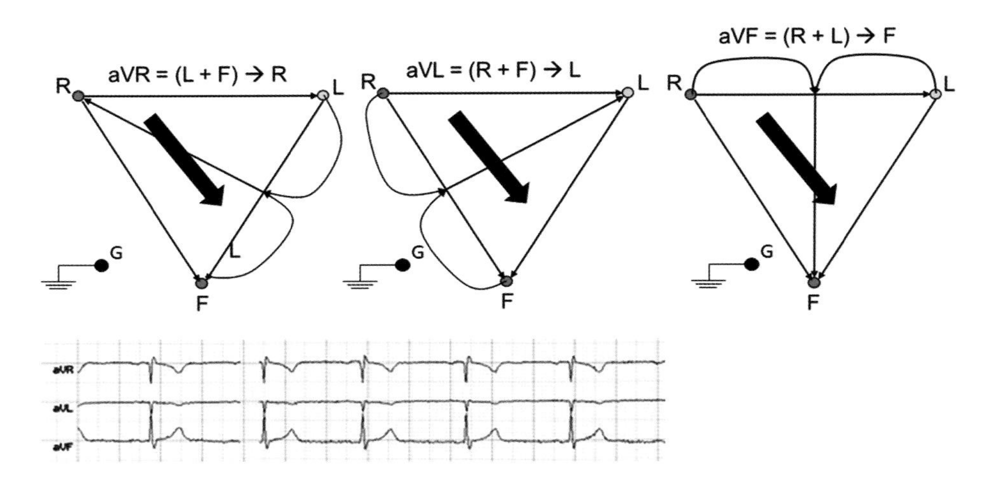

Figure 2.10 The electrical heart vector (black arrow) and its vector relation of the augmented voltage lead according to Goldberger aVR, aVL, and aVF, which influences the ECG amplitude and orientation.
Source: J. Güttler

movement (REM) phase, and the EEG for the deep sleeping phase [71]), or for neurological diagnosis (to identify epilepsy, etc.). As can be seen in Figure 2.11, the EEG electrode placement is more complex compared to the six-channel ECG (shown in Figure 2.8). The electrodes (A1 and A2) on the earlobe represent the reference electrodes. The other electrodes measure toward A1 and A2, whereas the electrodes placed on the left hemisphere of the head correspond to A1, and the electrodes placed on the right side of the hemisphere correspond to A2.

However, also in the field of the EEG, a lot research focuses on the brain computer interface (BIC), which aims to control computer by thoughts. The BIC devices are already on the market; however they are not designed to control the computer but instead to allow further research on it. They consist of active electrodes (and much fewer electrodes, because here a 19-channel investigation is less important), which allow for dry measurement and measurement through the hair. The active electrodes also exist for the ECG, which allow an easier implementation into the home environment. However, active electrodes are very sensitive and unfortunately catch more noise easily. Therefore, it may also easily happen that eye movements disturb EEG measurement.

2.3 Basic Knowledge in the Fields of Geriatrics, Sociology, Etc.

As mentioned in Chapter 1, not only is the old age itself the cause of the problems, but also the multimorbidity and the resulting diseases, which reduce the quality of life and

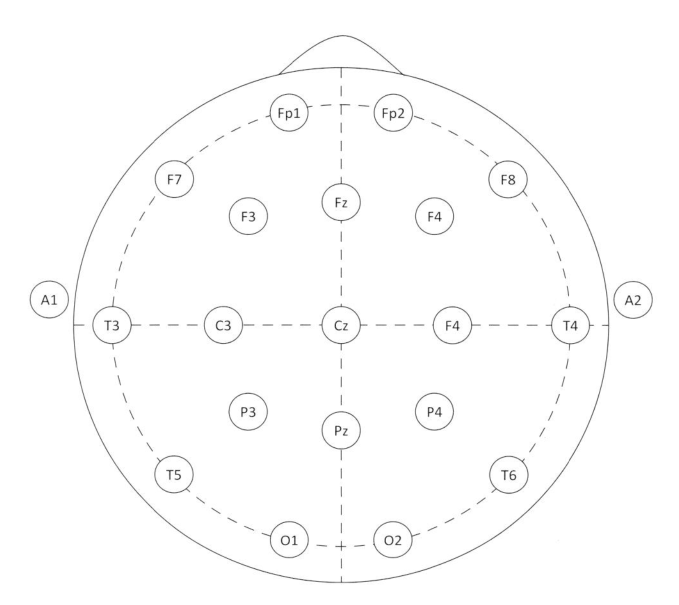

Figure 2.11 Schematic electrode placements for an EEG with 19 channels.
Source: J. Güttler

potentially lead to death. In Chapter 1, it was also mentioned that aging is not programmed, but it is an evolutionary result. In this chapter, a more detailed explanation of what exactly happens when we age, as well as what typical diseases are awaiting the aging person (and causes multimorbidity) is provided. Also, aspects of possible prevention will be discussed for the briefly summarized diseases.

The prevention aspects of the diseases mentioned in this chapter are of major importance for AAL because it is by them that life quality and the work force for the society remain preserved. Considering the social development (see Section 1.2) which showed that the number of elderly will increase while at the same time the population of young people will decrease by 2050, it is envisaged that there will be much higher retirement ages. Therefore, to keep the quality of life and the work force that the future generation of seniors can sustain for the predictably extended work life, early prevention is a key part of AAL, and must consequently involve the young generation.

Although aging is not programmed in the genes, the genes definitely have an impact on the aging progress. A very rare disease, which proves this theory, is called progeria [2]. Progeria is a disease caused by gene defects and affects DNA repair mechanisms, replication abilities, or the chromatin structure. Progeria can be differentiated into different kinds, Wiedemann–Rautenstrauch syndrome, Hutchinson–Guilford progeria syndrome, Werner syndrome, etc. However, all these kinds of progeria are segmental, which means that the different aspects of the (accelerated) aging process are differentially accelerated. The life expectancy is reduced to ~20 years, because of the age-related fragility, disease, and multimorbidity, which already start in childhood.

According to [2], genes influence roughly one-fifth up to one-third of the aging process. The other influencers consist of environmental factors (toxins, radiation, health nutrition, etc.) and happenstance. The telomere at the end of the chromosomes, for example, are known as the "biological clock." With each cell separation, the telomeres become shorter, until they are nearly vanished. In that case, the cell loses the ability to replicate (i.e., to replace another cell). These cells are called senescent cells. Depending on the cellular stress (which means, how often a cell in a specific tissue must be replaced because of environmental factors), the time it takes a telomere to shorten changes. The more often and faster the cells must replicate, the faster the telomeres become shorter. Other additional known reasons of the aging process at the cellular and molecular level, according to [2], include:

- Antioxidant protection mechanism;
- Amount of senescent cells;
- Accumulation of wrong processed or damaged proteins;
- Accumulation of mutations, especially with mDNA;
- Modification of the hormonal metabolic regulations, especially of the hormone Insulin/IGF.

Because of environmental factors like toxins and nutrition intake, etc., and the metabolic speed, the body, or organs, must replace cells in different amounts and frequency. This leads to different accelerations of the aging process from individual to individual, or even from organ to organ of the same individual.

Von Zglinicki [2] described the physiological changes while aging as follows: at the beginning, there are related function restrictions only noticeable under stress. The functional changes of the heart lead to a reduced exercise capacity. The reduced protection mechanism leads to an increased susceptibility to infections in the lungs, or to a higher aspiration risk (because of a too weak cough reflex). Additionally, by the loss of functionality of B- and T-lymphocytes (immune cells of the specific immune system, which offers the main protection for an individual in a specific climate area), the susceptibility to infections, cancer, and autoimmune processes are increased. The functionality of the kidneys and the metabolic activity of the liver are also reduced. Hormonal and neuronal steering and regulation processes are also changing and lead to different sleeping rhythms, reduced reaction time, and memory disorders. The changes in bone structure increase the probability of fractures. The reduction of the capability of the sensory organs and at the same time reduction of muscle strength increase the risk of accidents. Finally, the skin is also affected. The subcutaneous tissue including the capillary vessels and sweat glands are reduced leading to a reduction of sweat and fat production, as well as to a slowed down healing process. The turgor (inner cell pressure) and pigmentation (caused by degenerated skin cells) are also reduced leading to the typical look of the aged skin.

As it can be seen, the aging process leads to a continuously increased fragility, which sooner or later leads to unavoidable age-related diseases. The chosen diseases are introduced and briefly discussed since they are triggered by the factors mentioned in this section and lead to the reduced quality of life.

2.3.1 Metabolic Syndrome

The cardiovascular diseases are a summary of several heavy diseases. Mostly, these diseases start with the metabolic syndrome (also called the deadly quartet). According to [72], the deadly quartet consists of obesity, glucose intolerance (e.g., by Type II diabetes, see Section 2.3.3), hypertriglyceridemia (metabolic disorder of high blood level of triglycerides, which is a specific body fat), and hypertension (high blood pressure). The main trigger of this deadly quartet is obesity, which leads to hypertension and hyperinsulinemia (often occurring in Type II diabetes).

Therefore, [72] proposed that prevention of obesity has a larger impact than exercising, antihypertensive drugs and dieting. The metabolic syndrome occurs mostly in industrialized nations, which allowed the conclusion that this disease is triggered mainly by less activity and wrong nutrition intake. Sweet drinks like soda seem to support the obesity process very strongly, according to [73]. Additional to the physical activity and the food/drinking behavior, a too little/inefficient sleep schedule supports the development of obesity too [74]. Of course, it would be too easy to think that all obese people can improve their life quality by improving their daily habits. However, other factors influence obesity as well, genetic aspects, several diseases, side effect of some drugs, etc. Nevertheless, physical and mental activity with healthy food/drink and adequate sleep behavior strongly support the prevention of obesity.

The main issue on the metabolic syndrome and the following diseases is that they are largely symptom free. As soon as the first symptoms occur, it is mostly too late to rescue the life quality of the affected. Therefore, wearables are fast entering the public market, because they support people who are already actively preventing these age-related diseases. However, a weak point of wearables is that they work properly only if worn nearly always, which can quickly become inconvenient for the user. Therefore, a new approach in the research of AAL is the unobtrusive implementation of sensors for unobtrusive health analysis, which enables a seamless health check record, even if the wearables are sometimes not used (as already mentioned in Section 1.1).

2.3.2 Consequences of the Deadly Quartet

If someone is ignoring the result of the AAL devices, or is generally not screening his health status, the metabolic syndrome will lead to more serious diseases. Mainly, high blood pressure will damage the vessel walls of the arteries, leading to the development of occlusions (also known as stenosis). Depending on the region of the affected vessel, different diseases start, e.g., the peripheral artery disease. Commonly, legs are more affected than arms. The undersupply by a thrombus leads to pain while walking (also called claudication), and later to permanent pain in the affected extremity. If no improvement by medical treatment occurs soon, ulcers/gangrenes occur, meaning open wounds which are not healing/closing anymore. Sometimes it can happen that the thrombus is losing from the vessel wall and this leads to an embolus. If the embolus enters smaller arteries, an acute limb ischemia can be triggered (sudden stop of blood flow) [75]. If this condition stays untreated, the affected will lose the extremity by tissue necrosis.

Of course, the veins can also suffer under the metabolic syndrome. However, if here an occlusion is growing, the situation is even more dangerous than in the peripheral artery disease. This disease is also known as phlebothrombosis. While the affected extremity is normally white and cold in an acute limb ischemia, here the affected extremity seems blue and hot, and the skin is under great tension. Of course, here also, the affected can lose the whole extremity. However, it can also happen again that the thrombus will break lose from the vessel walls and become an embolus. Although the phlebothrombosis vanishes, this is a very dangerous life situation, because the embolus will pass the right heart atrium and ventricle, and enter the small blood circulation. As soon as the embolus enters the pulmonary artery, a lung embolus starts, which can end lethally. In [76], it is mentioned that between phlebothrombosis and the possible resulting pulmonary embolism much evidence exists that obesity increases the risk of disease.

If the occlusion is occurring in the coronary artery, this disease is called coronary artery disease, or myocardial infarction (also known as heart attack). Beside the metabolic syndrome, the risk of disease on a heart attack can additionally increase by stress, left ventricular hypertrophy, total cholesterol, and smoking [77]. Finally, also the vessels for the brain supply can be affected, which leads to a stroke (also known as cerebrovascular accident/insult). Here also, smoking additionally increases the risk of diseases on a stroke. The metabolic syndrome mainly increases the risk for an ischemic stroke. However, intracerebral hemorrhage is also possible, e.g., as a result of a ruptured aneurysm. However, for strokes, the ischemic strokes are dominant [78]. In both cases (heart attack and stroke) there is a similar pathomechanism; the blood supply to the heart or brain tissue behind the occlusion (caused by a thrombosis or embolus) is interrupted leading to a necrosis of the affected heart or brain cells. This first reduces the function of the affected organ, and finally leads to the death of the affected person. According to the [79], the main statistical reasons for death are listed in Table 2.1.

As it can be seen in Table 2.1, chronic ischemic heart disease, which can be seen as secondary diseases of the deadly quartet, is the number one reason of death. However, not only is the number one related to the metabolic syndrome, but also numbers two, four, seven, and ten. Counting the amount of dead people together gives an impression of the real victims of the deadly quartet.

2.3.3 Diabetes Mellitus

Type II diabetes (also called adult-onset diabetes), is totally different from Type I diabetes, and theoretically curable. Type I diabetes is an autoimmune disease, where the immune system attacks the islets of Langerhans of the pancreas. The islets of Langerhans (also known as pancreatic islets) are responsible for the endocrine function (i.e., the production of insulin and its injection into the blood). Once the immune system has destroyed all islets of Langerhans, insulin production stops, and if untreated, will lead to death. Fortunately, by frequently using injections of the insulin hormone, the

Table 2.1 Death Reasons according to ICD-10 in 2014 [79]

Number	Death Reason	Died	
		Amount	Share in %
1	Chronical ischemic heart diseases	69,890	8.0
2	Acute myocardial infarction	48,181	5.5
3	Lung cancer	45,049	5.2
4	Heart insufficiency	44,551	5.1
5	Other chronical diseases	27,008	3.1
6	Dementia	24,867	2.9
7	Hypertensive heart diseases	22,859	2.6
8	Breast cancer	17,804	2.1
9	Colon cancer	16,899	1.9
10	Stroke	16,753	1.9

diseases can be treated (although not cured) and the life expectancy of the diseased is nearly unchanged. People suffering from Type I diabetes are mostly very slim, as insulin is not only responsible for the absorption of sugar into the cells, but also stops the transfer of fat into sugar. As Type I patients do not produce insulin, fat gets immediately transferred to sugar by biological processes in the cells. Being an autoimmune disease, genetics are mainly responsible for the disease. However, the immune system is normally triggered mostly by unknown environmental factors.

Type II diabetes is completely different. The islets of Langerhans operate normally. This means that the affected patients produce insulin. However, the cells of the affected are oversaturated with sugar and start to ignore the hormone (i.e., Type II diabetes is an insulin resistance disorder) [80]. This leads to a vicious cycle, because at the beginning, the body compensates this problem by producing more insulin until the cells react. However, this will increase the insulin inhibition of the cells. Sooner or later, there is permanent insulin in the blood, which also permanently stops the transfer of fat into sugar. This then means that each gram of fat will be stored, and this is what finally leads to obesity. The high sugar concentration in the blood additionally changes the osmotic pressure, the liquid of the cells gets into the vessels and leads finally to an increased blood pressure. This pathomechanism leads again to the metabolic syndrome as already explained in Section 2.3.1. The use of insulin injections, as it is used in Type I diabetes, is only a patchwork to reduce the sugar concentration in the blood, but it also supports the obesity process.

Nevertheless, Type II diabetes is curable by lifestyle change. The same prevention as described at the beginning of Section 2.3 is necessary. Diet (especially the reduction of sugar consumption), until the metabolism of the body is recovered, and less sugar intake compared to the normal behavior, combined with appropriate physical activity, could cure the disease. G. Herold [81] expressed that body weight normalization can avoid or at least slow down the progress of Type II diabetes.

Unfortunately, in industrialized nations, the diseased person, sooner or later, will use insulin or other medication.

2.3.4 Osteoporosis

Osteoporosis, a disease of the bone structure, consists of two main features: reduced bone density and bone quality (i.e., increased fragility) [82]. The bone marrow fills the human bones, but in the regions where no bone marrow fills the bones, normally a spongy bone structure is found. This structure allows a highly robust, yet very light bone architecture. If the bones would consist only of compact bone substance, the body weight would significantly rise. This lightweight construction of the bone structure allows that just 15 percent of the human body weight is caused by the bone structure.

The bones are permanently rebuilt. While osteoblasts construct the bone, osteoclasts destruct the bone structure. This allows the bones to adapt to the environment, e.g., increasing bone substance if necessary, or decreasing if the person is too inactive. For example, if an astronaut is in the space, the muscle and bone structure decreases, because of the missing forces on the tissue (caused by the weightlessness) [83]; gravity is a necessary stimulation to increase the bone density. Also, in old age the bone structure is slightly reduced, which is also one reason why it is easier for the elderly to break a bone. However, if the bone structure decreased significantly, the affected become highly fragile (osteoporosis called). A typical break point is the femoral neck.

In most people, the exact reasons triggering primary osteoporosis are unknown. It is assumed that postmenopausal estrogenic absence is an important factor in osteoporosis development [84], which is one reason why females are more often affected than males. Secondary osteoporosis is mainly caused by influenceable factors, hyperthyroidism, steroid therapy, Type II diabetes, very sweet drinks with acid (sodas), heavy caffeine or chocolate consumption, smoking, fashion trends like thigh gaps and slimness, etc. [82], [85].

However, other factors can also trigger this disease, disturbed cortisone, or calcium metabolism, lack of sex hormones (in males), Type I diabetes, lactose intolerance, chronic indigestions, etc. In young age, the disease can nearly be cured by changing the lifestyle through training, avoiding nicotine, reducing fall risk (prevention of fractures, which would lead to immobilization) and medicine (calcium, vitamin D [82], osteoclast-disturbing drugs, etc.). However, the disease progression can only be slowed down, or stopped, but the existing damage on the bone structure cannot be fully reversed.

Osteoporosis leads also to a typical shape, which is caused by broken vertebral bodies. The typical "s" shape of the spinal column is amplified, while at the same time the body height is reduced. The stomach gets shifted to the front and a humpback grows (see Figure 2.12).

2.3.5 Parkinson's Disease

Parkinson's disease normally starts around 50 years of age (or older). However, there is a minority who become affected much earlier (from 30 years of age) [86]. Furthermore, in cases where the disease is inherited, it starts earlier (~40 years of age). This disease is

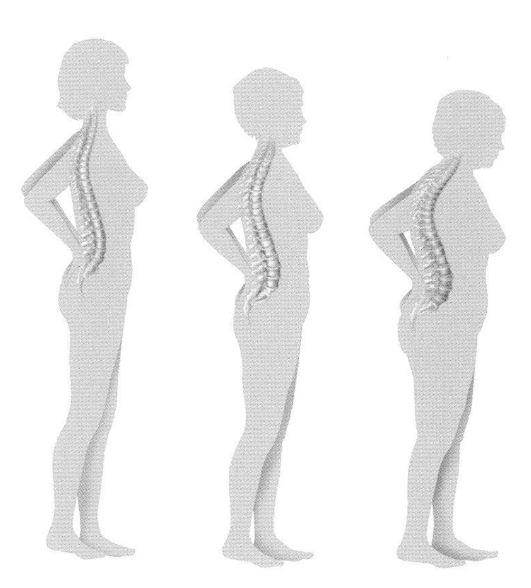

Figure 2.12 Schematic representation of age-related shaping of the spinal column, and its age-linked body shape and osteoporosis.
Source: BSIP/UIG via Getty Images

becoming more prevalent due to demographic changes (see Section 1.2). Pesticides and posttraumatic occurrences, infections, and misused drugs are other known causative possibilities. However, the reason for developing Parkinson's disease is mostly unknown. The pathomechanism is as follows; loss of nerve cells of the substantia nigra, which is an area located in the brainstem and responsible for the production of dopamine hormone, in the diseased leads to a lack of dopamine. The first symptoms occur as soon as significant dopamine levels are missing in the blood.

The cardinal symptoms are: tremor (usually rest tremor), rigidity (also known as lead-pipe or cogwheel symptom), akinesia (or bradykinesia), as well as the loss of postural reflexes [87]. However, other symptoms, e.g., blister disorder, visual disorder, sensory disorder, sexual dysfunctions, sleep disorder, and psychological changes can occur while the disease progresses. Typical symptoms include gait disturbance, sparely gesture and mimic, small handwriting and dysarthria (disorder of the speech motor activity).

Parkinson's disease belongs to the degenerative nerve diseases, which cannot be cured. Dopamine injections have no curing effect, as the blood-cerebral barrier filters this hormone. Fortunately, the pre-stage of dopamine, called L-Dopa [88] (levodopa), can pass the blood-cerebral barrier and thereby enter the brain. This drug at least slows down the disease progression. The use of deep brain stimulation can additionally reduce the symptoms, however, it is dangerous, as needle electrodes must be inserted through the healthy brain areal up to the substantia nigra. Nevertheless, these interventions do not stop the progression of the disease but can only slow down the disease and eventually the affected becomes hospitalized.

2.3.6 Dementia

Dementia is a collective word for several diseases of the brain. One of the most well-known diseases increasingly becoming more prevalent because of an aging population is Alzheimer's disease. Here, the brain (especially the hippocampal region) is affected mostly by underdevelopment [89]. This degeneration is caused by the collapse of several axons of the nerve cells. The embedded tau protein then produces plaques. The plaques, additionally, disturb the signal transmission on the remaining functional synapses.

The reduced volume of the gray tissues, which mainly are the processing nerve cells, while the white nerve tissues are mainly responsible for information transmission. Additionally, the ventricles are enlarged, causing a reduction of the brain volume.

The main known symptom is memory reduction (especially the short-term memory), but also disorders of orientation and time perception are usual symptoms. The practical skills are limited, and the communication abilities reduced. Unfortunately, for Alzheimer's disease, there exists no cure. The progression of Alzheimer's or other dementia diseases can be slowed down by some drugs (e.g., acetylcholinesterase) and by cognitive training. In [90], it is even mentioned that cognitive training should be used to prevent Alzheimer's as early as possible. The prognosis of Alzheimer's disease is that within six years (on average) the affected will die [91].

2.3.7 Sensory Organs: Eyes and Ears

In addition, our sensory organs also suffer during aging; it doesn't matter how good the eyes of a person are, the eyes seem to get weaker with age (Presbyopia). The reason is that the accommodation strength (i.e., the variable optical refraction power of the eye) of the lenses is reduced since the older a person becomes, the more the water in the core of the lenses reduces. This further leads to reduced elasticity and is the reason for the reduction in accommodation strength. For example, young people have an accommodation ability of 14 dpt, while a person of ~45 years has only 3 dpt left [92].

Some elderly may have bad luck, e.g., by a disturbed metabolism. If glucose crystals get stored in the lenses, the liquid will be bounded to the crystals resulting in secondary cataracts. Here, a predisease (e.g., Type II diabetes) triggers this condition. Of course, the standard cataract can occur without diabetes, and may be caused, e.g., by X-ray, ultraviolet light, electric current, and also punch or stab injuries. A cataract is characterized by the swelling and clouding of the lenses [93] (which changes the image recognition of the human eye as depicted in Figure 2.13). These events finally lead to complete blindness of the affected eye. Although it is possible that only one eye is affected by a cataract, the second eye, sooner or later, also becomes affected. A cataract is curable by replacing the diseased lens with an artificial lens.

A more serious disease is glaucoma. In this disease, the drain-away of the anterior chamber is blocked leading finally to very high intraocular pressure. The result is that the nerve cells on the retina suffer from the two large intraocular pressures, which leads to disturbance in image recognition (see Figure 2.14), as well as blindness in the end

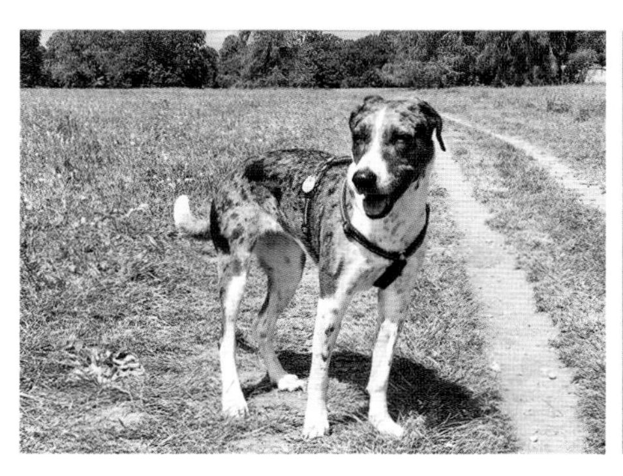
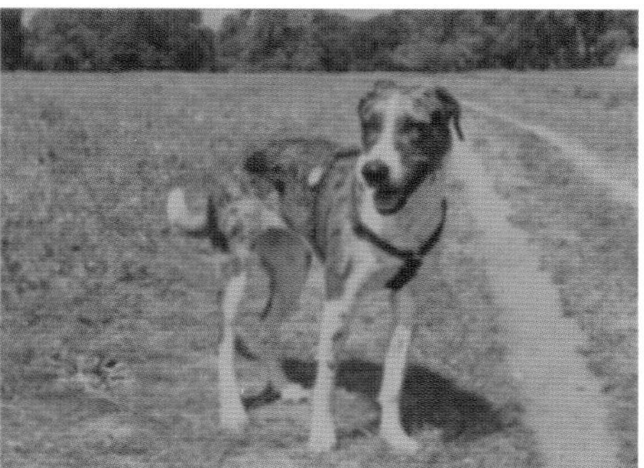

Figure 2.13 Left: an image as seen by a normal person.
Source: Schlandt
Right: the same image as seen by a person with a cataract.
Source: Schlandt, Image produced using the "Vision and Hearing Impairment Simulator," available from www.inclusivedesigntoolkit.com

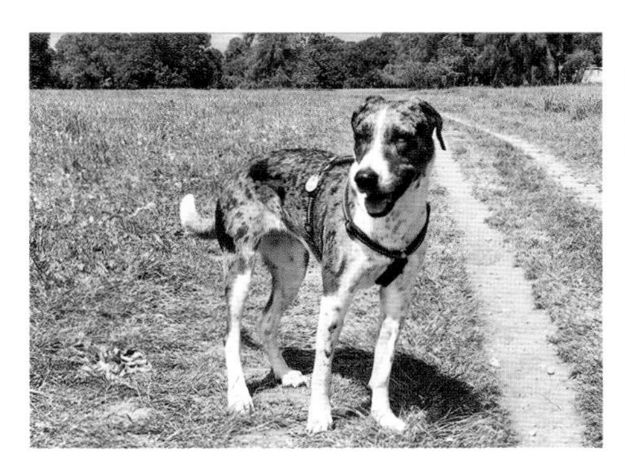
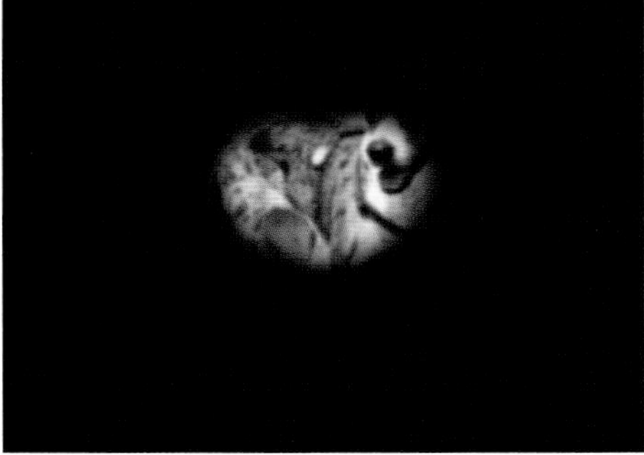

Figure 2.14 Left: an image as seen by a normal person.
Source: Schlandt
Right: the same image as seen by a person with glaucoma.
Source: Schlandt, Image produced using the "Vision and Hearing Impairment Simulator," available from www.inclusivedesigntoolkit.com

stage [94]. Ignoring secondary glaucoma triggered by infections or traumata, glaucoma is distinguished as either open-angle or closed-angle glaucoma. In closed-angle glaucoma, the angle between the cornea and iris is too narrow (e.g., due to thick lenses), so that the liquid within cannot drain (via Schlemm's canal). In open-angle glaucoma, the drain-away is blocked directly by degenerative changes in the Schlemm's canal, or to be more precise, at the surrounding trabecular meshwork. Medication is available for the regulation of the ocular pressure, and another treatment option today is the use of LASER to create an artificial drain-away canal.

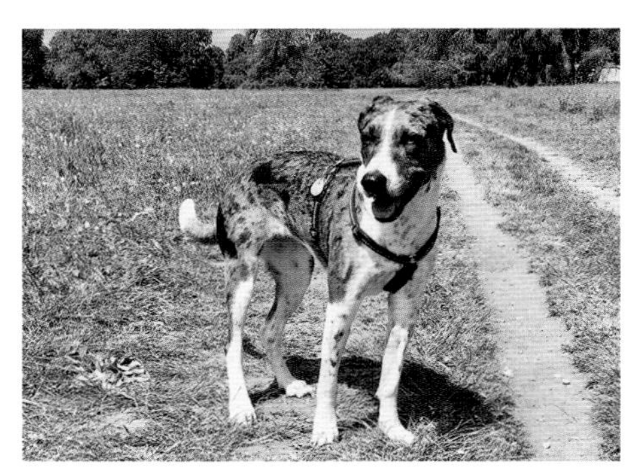

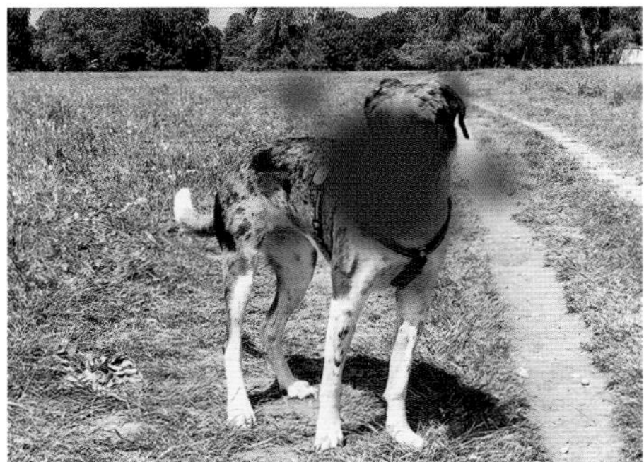

Figure 2.15 Left: an image as seen by a normal person.
Source: Schlandt
Right: the same image as seen by a person with age-related macular degeneration.
Source: Schlandt, Image produced using the "Vision and Hearing Impairment Simulator," available from www.inclusivedesigntoolkit.com

Even more serious is age-related macular degeneration. Generally, there are two different types of age-related macular degenerations existing: dry and wet [95]. Usually, affected people (up to 85% of the age-related macular degeneration) suffer from the dry version of the disease. Here, metabolic end products get deposited between the retinal pigment epithelium and the blood vessels (called drusen). This then leads to an undersupply of the nerve cells of the retina behind the drusen, resulting in necrosis of the affected retina tissue. When the macula lutea (yellow spot), which is the area on the retina where most nerve cells for visual reception exist (i.e., where the lens focus the light, so that a human can see sharp), is affected, the diseased person loses visual acuity (see Figure 2.15).

Additionally, up to ~15 percent of macular degeneration patients suffer from wet macular degeneration complications. Here, the progression of the disease is accelerated by vessels that grow through the retina pigment epithelium, which supply the nerve cells with blood. Unfortunately, these vessels lead to an additional uplift of the retina pigment epithelium and are also more permeable than normal vessels (this causes fluids to entering into the interstitium and additionally support the lift up of the nerve cells of the retina). By LASER therapy (or alternative photodynamic or by antibodies), the progression of the wet macular degeneration can be slowed down. However, the disease progresses faster than the dry macular degeneration. In each patient, the disease progresses differently and normally affects both eyes.

According to the famous picture by La Fée Électricité in Musée d'Art Moderne de la Ville de Paris (from Raoul Dufy for the International Exhibition 1937), when the human environment became bright and loud due to electricity, Raoul Dufy let her run away, while the Fée Électricité covers her ears (visible on the left side of Raoul Dufy painting). Furthermore, besides the eyes, the ears also get weaker in old age, proving that Dufy was right with his painted prognosis that the future will become bright and (too) loud.

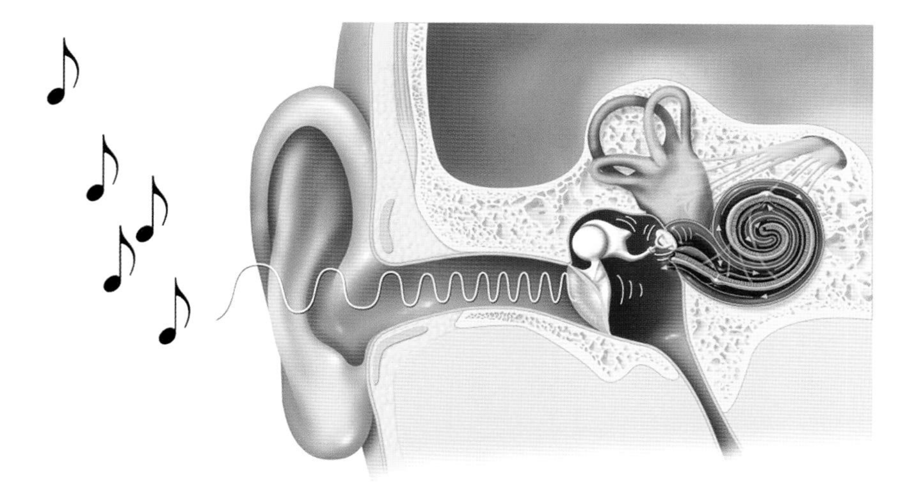

Figure 2.16 The tympanum and its connection to the cochlea via the hammer, anvil, and stirrup, which connects the ear drum and the oval window and enables mechanoelectrical transduction in the human ear.
Source: BSIP/UIG via Getty Images

People who live in very quiet areas (e.g., deserts) keep their hearing ability up to high age. The "natural" loss of hearing ability is frequency related. Newborns and children can hear in the range of frequencies from 16 Hz up to 16,000 Hz, however, the ability to hear at higher frequencies (>10,000 Hz) reduces with increasing age [96]. Age-related hearing loss (i.e., deafness and presbycusis), are a result of (or at least partially responsible for) chronic noise damage to the ears, i.e., from loud environments [97].

The ear can be split into three areas; outer, middle, and inner [97]. The middle and inner ear consist of the interface which converts a mechanical air pressure wave into an electrical signal (also called mechanoelectrical transduction) via the eardrum, which is the smallest bones in the human body, hammer, anvil, stirrup (middle ear), and the cochlea (inner ear in combination with nerves). In the cochlea (see Figure 2.16), hair cells get stimulated by the tectorial membrane after getting into oscillation through the basilar membrane. The basilar membrane triggers the tectorial membrane by the traveling wave triggered by the oval window (also visible in Figure 2.16), which is the interface to the stirrup.

According to the tube of the cochlea and its resonance frequency characteristics, only the hair cells (which belong to the corresponding frequency) on a specific spot get stimulated. These hair cells then translate the mechanical pressure wave into an electrical signal. If the middle ear gets destroyed because of disease (the eardrum is broken, etc.), the person loses their hearing ability. However, if the hearing capability via bone conduction is unchanged good. If the hair cells are destroyed because of exposure to extensively loud sounds over a long period of time, e.g., loud music, then the hearing ability suffers from air and bone conduction.

However, the bone conduction allows to bypass the middle ear and to send sound directly to the inner ear [97]. A common area to place a hearing aid, which is working via bone conduction, is the mastoid. Of course, in case the inner ear is damaged, the hearing aid via bone conduction does not improve the hearing abilities compared to hearing via air conduction. Hearing aids consist basically of a microphone, a microchip responsible for capturing the audio signal and forwarding to a loudspeaker that emits the sound via an amplifier, and a battery as a power source. By using an implemented interface, hearing aids for bone conduction forward the sound directly to the bones of the skull via the mastoid.

3 Built Environment Upgrading for AAL (BeuAAL)

As society ages, the building stock needs to be upgraded. A proper Ambient/Active Assisted Living (AAL) implementation needs a holistic approach; consequently, the environment itself needs to be adapted to the new needs of its inhabitants. Spatially and functionally, homes, and generally the built environment, may not meet the requirements of the elderly anymore. Demographic changes and the effects of an aging society also affect buildings and the built environment. Rapid refurbishment processes, quick adaptation protocols, and appropriate maintenance procedures become a necessity in order to not disturb the elderly and provide them with comfortable and functional homes and spaces. This is the main motivation behind the message of this chapter, which deals with the issue of how to adapt the living built environment for the elderly by use of fast and unobtrusive procedures. Moreover, a method for the assessment of strategies for built environment upgrading for AAL (BeuAAL) in early stages is presented. This chapter will help encouraging several stakeholders to accomplish building renovations for the elderly using robotics and automated tools.

3.1 Why Upgrade Existing Buildings and Homes for the Elderly?

The old built environment in an aging society is an issue that developed countries need to face. Decreases in population diminish the building market's potential, and especially in the real estate sector, the market is not as vigorous as when the population is growing and the main household types are families with children [98]. Currently, in developed countries, it is not as feasible to erect new buildings when compared to economically more expansive periods. However, it is also true that on average, older society members need more surface area per person to cover their requirements [99]. Two main issues will be dealt with next. First, an elderly person is more comfortable when living in a known environment, where the spatial ambience can easily be recognized (see Section 3.1.1). Second, research shows that renovation is a better choice than implementing a new building policy due to environmental issues such as land artificialization, material consumption, and recyclability (see Section 3.1.2).

3.1.1 Aging in Place

Research [100] shows that people late in life feel more comfortable, self-confident, better oriented, and less lonely if they remained where they lived as seniors, or at least lived in a place of their choosing. If there is a substantial change to an elderly person's living space, and especially if he or she doesn't accept it, the chances of quality of life deterioration and loss of health increase. It is better for the elderly to choose their built environment, or at least the residence, around which they feel most comfortable. But what if this built environment is not functional anymore for this person? Getting older might force a change in the elderly person's living scenario and sometimes require urgent responses. In some cases, the responses are minor modifications. Other times, major changes are necessary; an entire bathroom might need to be changed because it's not functional for the elderly user.

Normally, in terms of operability, the elderly need bigger bedrooms, bigger bathrooms, and adapted kitchens. However, on the other hand, compared to other types of households, lesser area is needed, because fewer residents live there. It seems obvious that a home conceived for hosting a traditional family with parents and children is not suitable for one or two people anymore. Though, especially in dense urban areas [101], there are economic feasibility issues for aging in place. When people get older and retire from their jobs, the pension they receive might not be enough to keep and maintain their former homes. In some cases, the elderly person might live alone. There are several options for maintaining the operative costs of the building and efficiently using a smaller income after retirement:

- If the housing market where the elderly person lives is expansive, or at least active, "reusing" and "reoccupying" the owner-occupied property is a good option [102].
- Currently, especially in big urban areas, the possibility of hosting a young person within the elderly house as a guest is a viable option.
- Cohousing for the elderly where people share part or the entire living space.

The first two options are good in an urban environment and when the real estate market demands new built surfaces. But if we are talking about rural regions where new home construction is not in demand, then some other options, such as cohousing, would be more appropriate.

Are building typologies and layouts adapted to these new ways of hosting elderly people? Is it easy to adapt a home in order to reach and meet the needs of the inhabitants? How could a home be adapted in a bespoke manner to meet the demands of the changing health conditions of the elderly? These questions will be answered in this chapter.

3.1.2 Environmental Issues Regarding Renovation

According to [103], renovating and refurbishing a building is more efficient compared to constructing a new one if we consider environmental issues. The main parameters are:

- Lower energy consumption. Building requires human activity that consumes more energy. However, building renovation needs much less energy than tearing down buildings and erecting new ones.

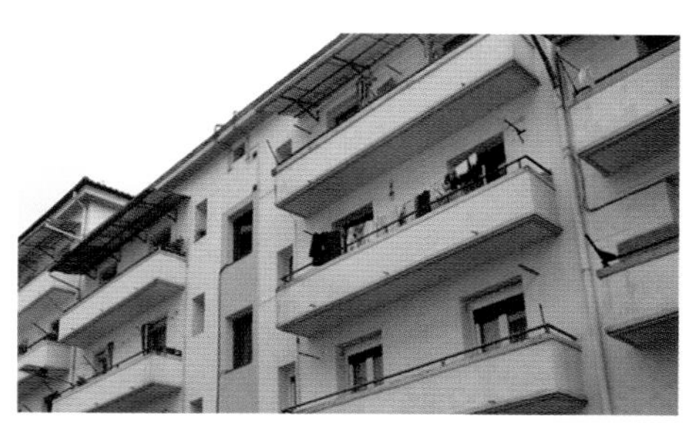
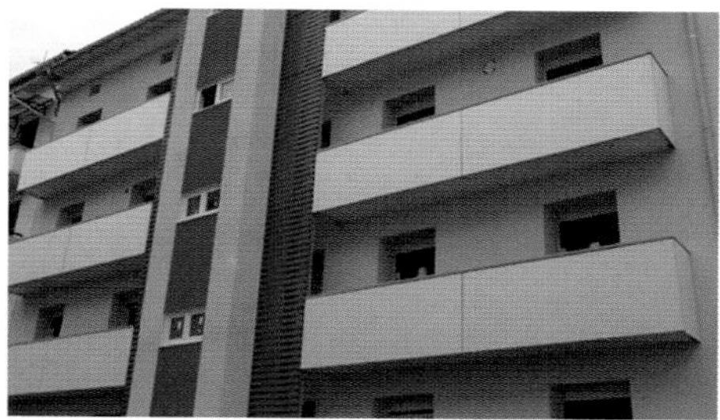

Figure 3.1 (left) Postwar era buildings, in particular, need to be upgraded for AAL implementation. In the Zenn project [106], manual procedures of refurbishment were undertaken (right) and the results are satisfactory according to the building users (Image by Debegesa).
Source: Debegesa

- Lower material consumption. A significant building renovation needs 60 percent less material than erecting a building with the same volume and surface area.
- Renovating is often more feasible than demolition and erection of a new building [104].

Therefore, some public administrations, such as the European Commission [105], are promoting building renovation as opposed to the policy of tearing down buildings and erecting new ones.

3.2 Parameters for a Comfortable AAL Built Environment

Advanced societies are following the trend of adapting their existing built facilities, cities, and infrastructures for better elderly life. Not only is the population getting older, but also the places where they used to live are no longer appropriate [107]. Many buildings, especially the ones built during the postwar era (Figure 3.1), were designed and erected following the criteria, regulation, economic feasibility, and household needs of that period. According to the main characteristics of the building stock [108], the problems that buildings and homes face regarding the senior population are:

- Inadequate thermal conditions. Elderly people are affected more by extreme weather conditions.
- Inadequate acoustic conditions. Noise in urban areas has increased compared to the postwar era, and the elderly suffer more as a result.
- Inaccessible spaces. In the postwar era there was often a lack of elevators and doorways with dimensions too narrow for a handicapped person. Kitchens, bathrooms, and bedrooms were not adapted.
- Improper lighting conditions resulting in an excess or lack of illumination.
- Unpleasantness of the built environment, where contact with vegetation is limited and social interaction is not possible.

These functional aspects of homes are not only for AAL implementation cases, but apply to general homes and buildings as well. Currently, the regulation and needs have become tighter than in the postwar era. However, the implementation of regulation is limited, but normally not compulsory. Economic feasibility is the main problem when upgrading buildings. It might be impossible to adapt some buildings as necessary due to technical and/or economic limitations.

Currently, and especially in the European Union, there are a number of research projects dealing with the optimization of renovation of existing buildings [105]. The majority of building renovation is focused on reducing energy consumption, i.e., one of the goals to achieve for the optimal AAL scenario. However, it´s not the only one; there are several other parameters to consider, as previously mentioned. Some of the parameters for a comfortable built environment will be further explained in the next section.

3.2.1 Thermal Comfort and Almost Zero Energy Consumption of the Built Environment

The elderly sometimes stay less socially active than the young [109]. Therefore, their homes and houses need to be thermally comfortable in order to avoid acquiring diseases related to high or low temperatures [110]. There are several ongoing public policies for adapting existing building stocks into thermally comfortable buildings that use very low energy [105]. For instance, the European Commission has set an objective for the year 2050: to minimize the energy consumption of buildings to nearly zero. The measures for reaching a nearly zero energy consumption in an existing building are diverse:

- Placing a highly insulating layer in the building envelope.
- Installing air-tight ventilation systems, mainly for cold temperatures. The outdoor–indoor air streams need to be prevented to keep a building thermally comfortable.
- Installing heat-recovery systems to ventilate an indoor space without losing heat.
- Installing new and efficient ventilations systems for heating and cooling.
- Installing energy collecting systems such as solar cells, water heating systems, and similar devices.
- Utilizing Renewable Energy Sources (RES) in building envelopes.

How can these advanced building skins and devices be installed in a rapid manner? Traditional installing techniques are long processes. As explained in Section 3.3, the unobtrusiveness of any kind of building renovation must always be considered when working on homes for the elderly. Besides passive measures for building renovation, there have been recent developments in the automated control of thermal energy and its storage [111] [112].

3.2.2 Acoustically Comfortable Built Environment

As already mentioned in Chapter 2, the elderly tend to stay at home, and it is therefore important that these spaces are noise-free, since the elderly are more sensitive to

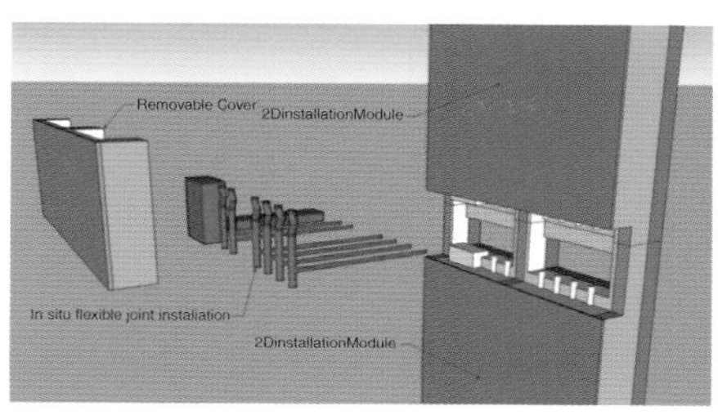

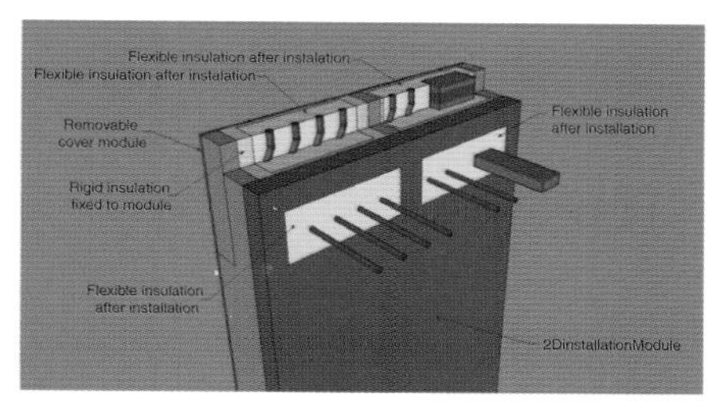

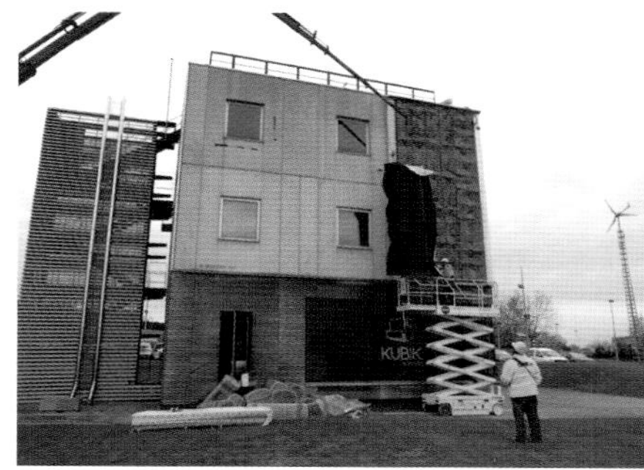

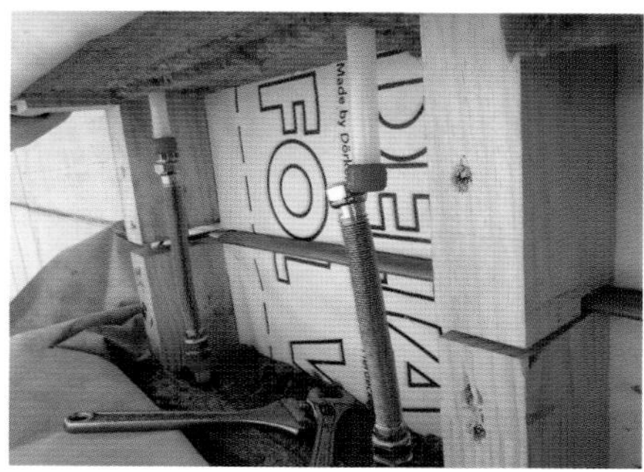

Figure 3.2 Prefabricated solutions for building thermal upgrading with services. BERTIM project [112]. The modules have a registrable part (left) at the point where services are connected to the interior of the existing building (center). These concepts were demonstrated in the Kubik building (right).
Source: BERTIM

unpleasant noise than the rest of the population. On the one side, the health condition of the elderly can be directly affected by noise; a noisy environment can increase the risk of stroke or other health problems [113]. On the other side, environmental perception can be disturbed by high noise. Therefore, the elderly cannot hear properly, especially at high frequencies, as mentioned in Section 2.3.7, which can contribute spatial disorientation.

In a home, there are two sources of noise: outdoor and indoor. On the one hand, noise can come from the building itself; neighbors and services generate noise within the building. For this purpose, internal wall and floor insulation is necessary, considering not only aerial noise, but also impact noise created by collision to the building's surfaces. On the other hand, noise sources often originate outdoors. There are two main solutions for the mitigation of outdoor noise. One is to adapt the existing buildings by using noise-insulating layers on the perimeters of homes. Some research projects have already dealt with the installation of prefabricated elements that can be installed in existing buildings (Figure 3.3) [114]. Another way is to contain the noise at the source, such as at highways, railways, and factories. Noise barriers are necessary at these points, especially in the surroundings of hospitals and care centers. To achieve this, it is recommended to use software tools developed for accurate noise detection and simulation, with which the necessary types of noise barriers can be foreseen (Figure 3.3) [115]. Finally, advanced materials and elements exist that facilitate the mitigation of noise and that can be installed in a few hours [116].

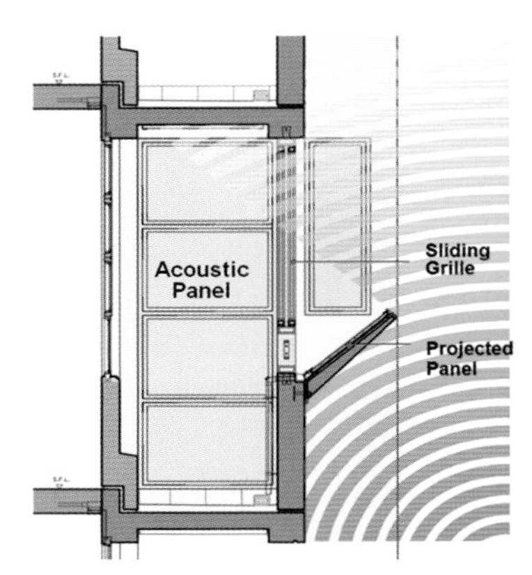

Figure 3.3 Use of prefabricated elements in existing balconies for indoor noise mitigation [114].
Source: Hong Kong Housing Department

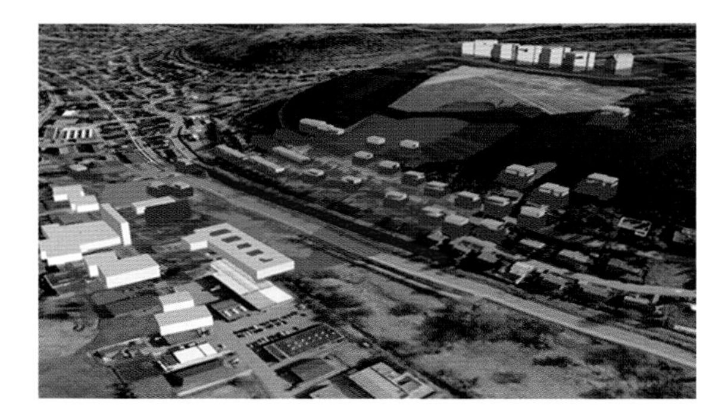

Figure 3.4 Noise simulation and prediction software noise3D [115].
Source: noise3D

Often, dangerous incidents occur on roads and railways. How do we design, manufacture, and install noise barriers fast without disturbing the traffic and the neighborhood? How do we achieve noise mitigation with automated devices and robotics? It is necessary to develop new technologies to answer these questions.

3.2.3 Accessible Built Environment for the Elderly

When the health conditions of an elderly person deteriorate, access to every location in the home becomes problematic. The active measures taken in the robotics field to address this issue will be explained in Section 4.6. Regarding the passive measures on the built environment, spaces might need to be changed. There are four major points to be considered:

- In the case of indoor areas, bathrooms, rooms, and kitchens are highly susceptible to major changes in order to become more accessible for the elderly.

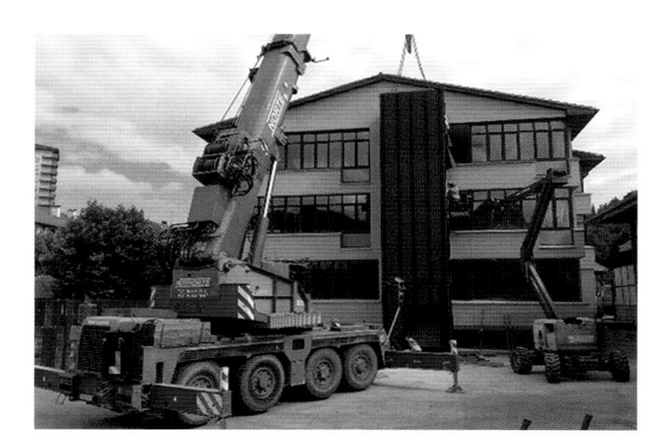

Figure 3.5 Installing a prefabricated elevator shaft. [117].
Source: EGOIN

- The elderly person may need assistance with bed-chair, chair-toilet and chair-bathroom transfers, depending on the person's health.
- In multistory buildings, elevators systems are needed to move incapacitated residents.
- Outdoor scenarios are more complex and varied, and thus they have bigger problems.

Currently, the installation of external elevators on existing buildings can be considered an automated operation. The elevator shafts can be prefabricated to as high as 12 meters, placed and fixed with the help of mobile cranes (Figure 3.5 left) [117]. Installing a prefabricated 3D module on existing buildings can be an option for creating accessible bathrooms for the elderly in old quarter buildings [118] (Figure 3.5, right).

3.2.4 Adequate Lighting for the Elderly

The elderly become more sensitive to lack of and/or excess lighting while aging. Proper natural and artificial lighting is necessary for the elderly in order to:

- Prevent accidents due to lack of lighting, especially in stairs, kitchens, and bathrooms. The AAL devices sometimes require adequate lighting for optimal functioning.
- Adapt the lighting to the biological clock and enhance comfortable visual situations. It has been tested and proved that techniques such as *Snoezelen* (controlled multi-sensory environment) are very helpful for people that suffer from dementia [119].

Both excess of light (too much sunlight) and lack of light affect the perception of objects. This can be a major problem when an elderly person needs to recognize food, for instance [120]. Fluorescent light diminishes the color spectrum of things. Therefore, the visual perception decreases [121]. This type of light should be avoided in homes for the elderly.

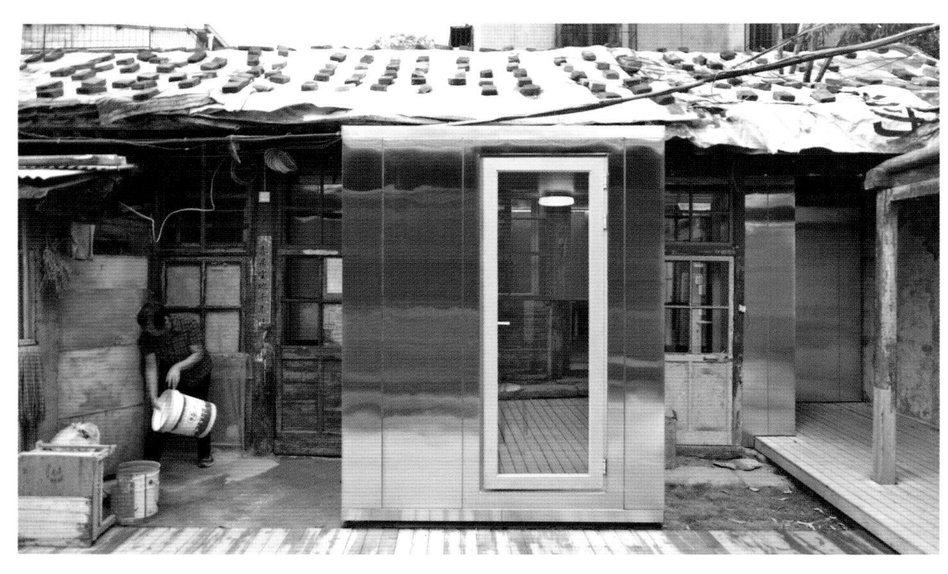

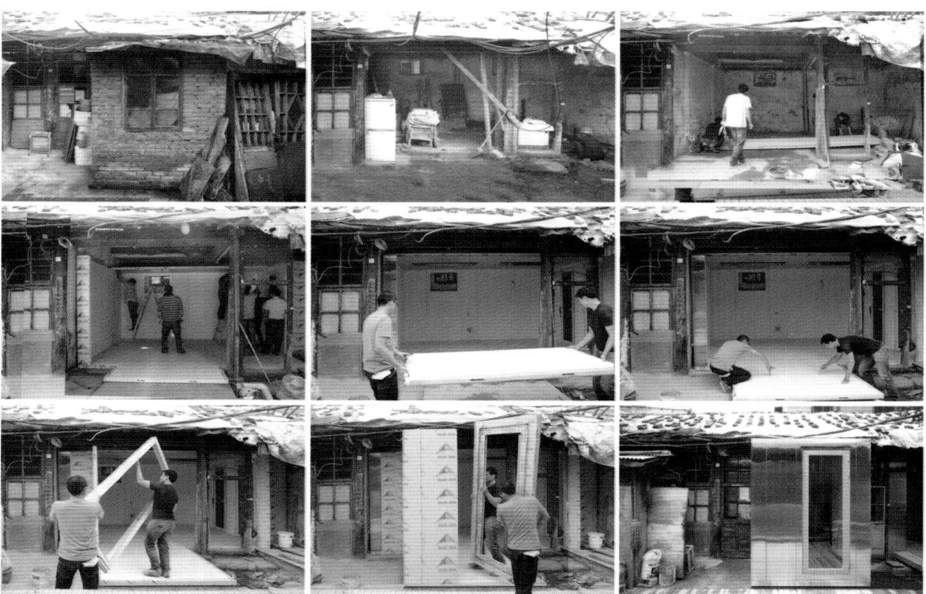

Figure 3.6 Prefab bathrooms and kitchens in an old Beijing quarter building [118].
Source: People's Architecture Office

3.2.5 A Green, Healthy, and Pleasant Built Environment for the Elderly

Many of the buildings erected during the postwar era followed very strict criteria regarding minimal house surface area. They were designed with many constrictions. Normally, these buildings were built very narrow and followed the trend of the period according to the "hygienist" criteria that preferred higher sun exposure in every corner

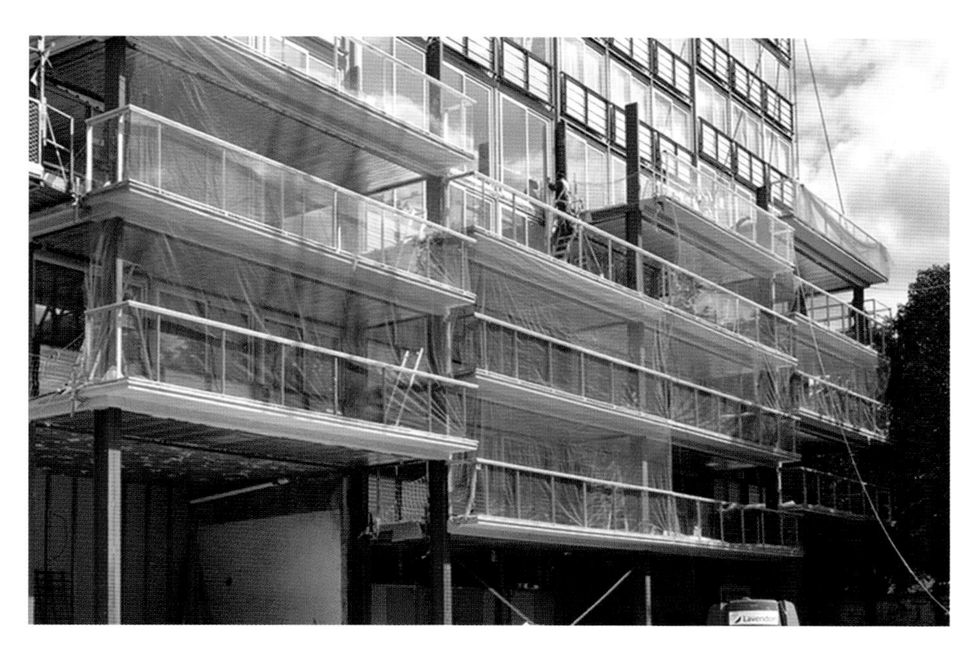

Figure 3.7 Building a new winter garden in the perimeter of the apartment building. A new pleasant area is added where there is a closer contact with the outdoor [123].
Source: Lacaton & Vassal

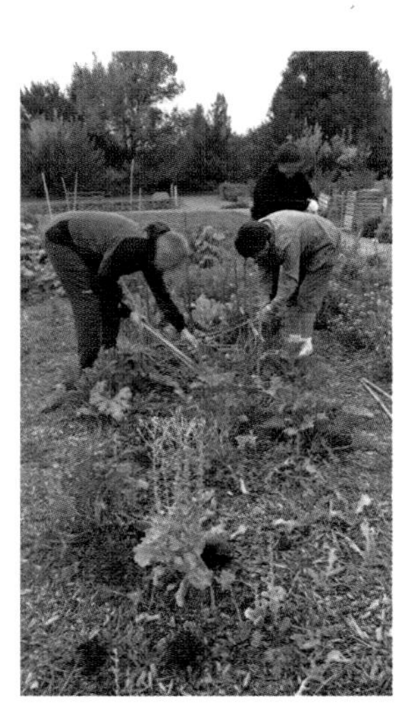

Figure 3.8 Community gardens for the elderly in urban areas.
Source: Jurgi Uriarte

of the apartment. The form, shape, lighting, color, and vegetation (or lack thereof) of a space can both positively and negatively stimulate an elderly's orientation, social interaction, and mobility [122].

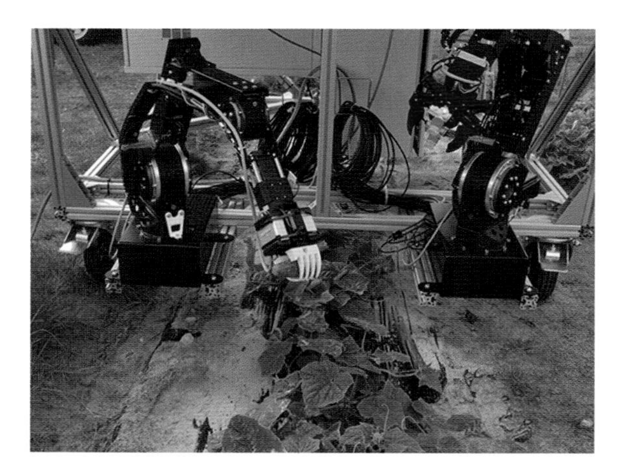

Figure 3.9 The CATCH project. Cucumber Gathering Green Field Experiments. EU FP7 research Grant Agreement no 601116 [125].
Source: Fraunhofer IPK

One interesting approach of enlarging apartments was carried out in Paris [123]. The project, as designed by Lacaton & Vassal architects, involved addition of a new interface room, similar to a winter garden (*jardin d'hiver*). Following the idea of the garden, it can be said that the members of a community can tighten their relations and improve their social life if they participate in common activities [124] (see Figure 3.8). Even though meeting around a garden is pleasant and healthy, not all elderly people have a health condition that allows for planting and harvesting. Agricultural robots can provide a solution for heavy works. Recent developments in robotics, such as the CATCH project, can be an option to properly maintain a garden for the elderly [125].

3.3 Parameters for an Unobtrusive BeuAAL through Automation and Robotics

Renovation works of a building are, traditionally, disturbing to the surrounding area. They generate noise, dust, and dirt. During renovation, depending on the amount of work, the inhabitants might be forced to leave their homes . The adaptation of a living space may be a major issue since the inhabitant may need to temporarily leave or suffer through the major renovation work. Therefore, there is a strong need to find new strategies for a more rapid installation process. Refurbishment works are annoying to building inhabitants and especially for the elderly. Therefore, some strategies are needed in order to minimize the negative effects of renovation of the built environment.

3.3.1 Maximize Off-Site Manufacturing and Minimize On-Site Works

Building upgrades often require the use of several materials, elements, and technologies. A minor renovation process might need to upgrade the structure, the distribution of services such as HVAC, water, ventilation, and ICT. Therefore, it is crucial to minimize in an orderly way the on-site execution of all these tasks. Currently, there is a trend of developing on-site robots using additive techniques or 3D printing [126]. This technology can be very useful in many fields, but for BeuAAL, these devices might be too slow, and also may generate dirt. Therefore, they may be too disturbing for a rapid and unobtrusive BeuAAL.

On the contrary, the prefabrication of modules might be a better option for rapidly installing and upgrading the devices for BeuAAL. As it has been deeply analyzed in previous volumes of Cambridge Handbooks on Construction Robotics [128], the prefabrication of buildings in the Japanese construction sector is highly developed. There is a long tradition of building with prefabricated modules, which (a majority of them) follow a strict and accurate modulation system based on the tatami system. This is an advantage for manufacturing and installing the modules. Moreover, this is also an important parameter for renovation. The Sekisui Heim [127] manufacturing company offers to their clients and the building owners a *long-term support system* with three main services:

- The maintenance and repair of the building elements, such as building structure. This is an important aspect in Japan due to earthquakes. The structures need to be kept in optimal conditions.
- Upgrading building elements and services in order to gain a better (energetic) performance.
- Upgrading the building to the owner's functional needs. The company is aware that the household's models are changing and the inner distribution as well as the accessibility of each of the areas has to be adapted to the new needs.

In the case of Sekisui Heim (Figure 3.10), the company offers its customers the possibility of a long-lasting building maintenance and an upgrading contract covering these three points.

3.3.2 Automated Tools and Robotic Devices for Building Upgrading

Robots are complex devices that need a long development process. Compared to a workshop or a factory, where the robot operates in a controlled environment, in building renovation, all these subsystems gain complexity. In order to operate, a robot for building renovation needs to fulfil at least three different requirements and subsystems:

- Robot body. This must be suitable to the built-environment. Bulky bodies must be avoided while stability must be preserved.
- End effector or end effector kit that operates several tasks.
- Control system. It must be synchronized with the sensing system for accurate positioning of the robot.

It might be clear to say that the existing industrial robots are not suitable, without being modified, to work on building renovation. The robots need to be readapted in order to safely reach every point of the built environment. Besides, the robots should work fast,

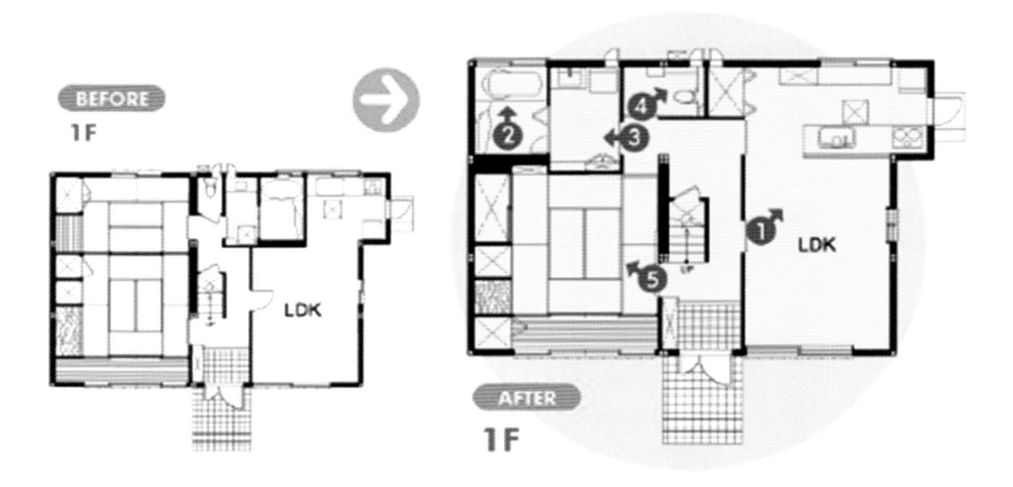

Figure 3.10 Example of rapid renovation process strategies by Sekisui Heim [127]. Source: Sekisui Chemical Co., Ltd.

accurately and flexibly without temporarily evacuating the residents. There can be two strategies for conceiving a robot for building renovation:

- Multiple synchronized single task and small robots.
- Unique unobtrusive body with a modular end-effector kit.

As an open question, it can be discussed whether the robotic system used for building upgrades could be merged with robots used for AAL.

3.3.3 Open Building Principles as Method for Gaining Flexibility

These buildings were conceived for serving certain types of inhabitants, mostly the traditional family household. Briefly, we can say that these were designed for young families. Today, these households are typically couples or individuals with older relatives. Since the elderly's physical and psychological conditions can vary with age, their home might consequently need to be periodically adapted. There are strategies that facilitate the change of the layout of the home. The Open Building concept and principles are based on a clear differentiation and hierarchization of the base building and the fit-out [129]. This principle permits a more flexible approach than the rigid-functionalism of buildings where the current layout and functionalities are too interdependent and not very flexible. A more independent approach could offer a more flexible layout and more functionalities. Related to this concept, there is the Axiomatic Design approach [130], in which the Independence Axiom has special relevance. This will be further explained in Section 3.4.

A good example of an Open Building was accomplished in Osaka in the project Next21 [131]. This building was conceived for the employees of the Osaka Gas company where there could be a rotation of building inhabitants.

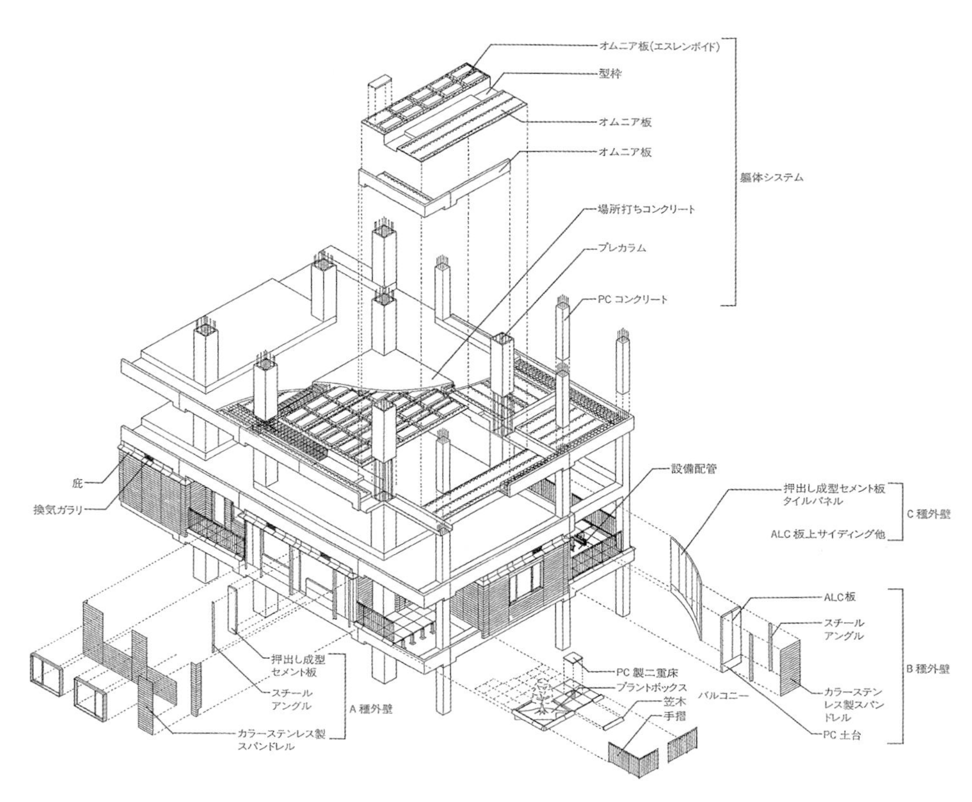

Figure 3.11 Next 21 Osaka project, based on Open Building principles [131].
Source: Shu-Koh-Sha Architectural and Urban Design Studio

3.4 Assessment of Early Strategies of BeuAAL

Within the European context, in the FP7 and H2020 research frameworks, the main building renovation research projects were focused on the energy-saving related topics [105]. However, in the future, it is expected that the trend will be diverted toward the renovation of homes (and built environment) considering AAL implementation [132]. An aging society requires the adoption of this strategy. *Built environment upgrading for AAL* is a concept that implies multihierarchized requirements and subsystems, where socioeconomic, environmental, and technologic aspects are related in micro- and macro scales. Achieving a complete AAL system requires cross-collaboration between partners of different fields. One problem is how to accurately assess a research project in its efficiency in facing the issues of AAL. Two types of stakeholders might need to enhance this situation. On the one hand, several public administrations are willing to implement AAL concepts. On the other side, technology developers are willing to market their output into the AAL. How can both organizations achieve the above goal successfully in a coordinated manner while considering human, environmental, and technological aspects? When developing a piece of technology, it is often necessary to

Table 3.1 Functional Requirements of the BeuAAL

First Level	Second Level
FR1: Comfortable AAL built environment	FR 1.1 Thermal comfort in zero energy consumption
	FR 1.2 Acoustic comfort
	FR 1.3 Accessible built environment for the elderly
	FR 1.4 Adequate lighting
	FR 1.5 Green built environment
FR2: Unobtrusive building upgrading	FR 2.1 Minimize on-site works
	FR 2.2 Automated tools and Robotic devices
	FR 2.3 Open building, flexibility

contextualize the approach with the existing trends and needs. The aim of this chapter is to establish a framework for guiding the preliminary stages of technology achievement of the so-called AAL and its built environment's management and upgrading.

This *built environment upgrading for AAL* concept can be broken down into many requirements and subsystems. How do we interrelate them in order to create a more cohesive system? The methodological approach presented in this chapter is meant to not only be a tool for the technology developers and companies, but also for the public administration. They will first check that the conceived and developed product or solution is suitable from a holistic perspective, considering human, environmental, and other technological perspectives. The technology for the building upgrading for AAL is not developed by a single centralized stakeholder, but by multiple, independent developers who push for their own achievements. Therefore, the technology developer needs to know if the proposed solution in the preliminary stages meets the needs of the so-called built environment upgrading for AAL. On the other hand, public administration will have the choice to contextualize each of the possible solutions with their aspects and to relate to them while defining policies and strategies. It has to be said that preliminary technology development is meant that the Technology Readiness Level (TRL) is 2 to 6 [133]. Besides, this methodology tool should be usable for both micro and macro scale systems of the built environment. For all the reasons explained, the remainder of this chapter will define a clear methodology for assessing Preliminary Stage Research Projects within the context of the built environment upgrading for AAL.

When installing technologies of AAL and upgrading an existing built environment, there is already a previously conformed physical constraint. The elderly person's home, house, neighborhood, city, and region comprise the environmental background. The BeuAAL strategies need to be adaptable to this background. The goal of the assessment is to check if a given research for BeuAAL meets the parameters and requirements mentioned beforehand in Sections 2.5.1 and 2.5.2. The assessment method is divided in two main steps as explained in Sections 3.4.1 and 3.4.2.

3.4.1 Formulation of the Functional Requirements and Qualitative Assessment

On the first step, the so-called Axiomatic design method for reorganizing the whole strategies for BeuAAL will be applied. As a short explanation of the Axiomatic Design, it can be said that there are four main, strongly interconnected domains: Customer domain, Functional domain, Physical domain, and Process domain. In the Customer domain, the Customer Attributes or needs are defined (CA). The Functional Requirements (FR) are part of the functional domain. In this domain, constraints such as economic feasibility are also underlined. The parameters seen in Sections 2.5.1 and 2.5.2 have been transformed to FRs within the Functional Domain.

Once is the achievement goals are known, the method to accomplish said goals must be discussed. The Physical domain is for conceiving the Design Parameters (DP) or physical artifacts. But is it feasible to achieve the adopted solution with regard to existing technologies? The DPs consist of a vast variety of solutions. These can correlate several scales of actuation; the micro-scale, such as a building or assistive apartment, or the macro-scale, such as smart transportation systems.

For relating the FR and the DP, a Design Matrix is used. The DPs can be considered as a set of solutions that fulfil the FRs. The objective of the matrix is to prove that the Independence Axiom is fulfilled, which means that each of the Design Parameters cannot interfere with the rest of the DPs and FRs. In other words, the Axiomatic Design will be used to define that the proposed solution and subsolutions do not interfere or are not contradictory to each other.

The technical feasibility of the DPs is checked on the Process Domain. Here, the Process Variables characterize the Design Parameters by introducing Production Process criteria. All the CAs, FRs, DPs, and PVs can be decomposed and hierarchized until a final, concrete, and feasible solution is set. A main matrix collects and correlates all the FRs and DPs. In the case of the AAL, the Main Matrix also correlates several Human-centered perspectives with purely technological solutions. Finally, for the development of the DPs, the so-called zig-zagging method is used.

This evaluation should be done during the conception of the technologic solution. It ensures that the technological solution must meet all requirements. If the technology fulfils this step, it can then be moved to the next step of assessment.

This AAL Functional Requirement Matrix must be flexible in terms of the novel socioeconomic and technological improvements. Furthermore, depending on the analysis of the needs and lacks of each moment and region, this system is subject to change.

3.4.2 Quantitative Assessment of Preliminary Technology Development for BeuAAL

In the second step, an evaluation of each of the DPs is necessary. This is used for gathering a quantitative aspect for defining the technology solutions and suitability within the BeuAAL concept. According to the Axiomatic Design, the Information Axiom states that the solutions with less content of information offer higher probability of success. This is definitely a statement for highly developed solutions, not for the first stages of a research project. For preliminary stages, a Multi-Criteria Decision Making (MCDM), such as COPRAS [134], model would guide the evaluation of preliminary technology development. In the case of multiple solutions, it would also be useful for deciding which of the possible solutions fit better within the same research project. In this subsection a list of attributes and indicators are presented to guide the future MCDM.

Table 3.2 Indicators of the BeuAAL in an Ideal Situation

Functional Requirements for BeuAAL (BeuAAL)		Attributes		
First Level	Second Level	Indicators	Direction	Weight(%) (wght)
FR1: Comfortable AAL built environment	FR 1.1 Thermal comfort in zero energy consumption	ΔT 21°C = 0	Min	12.5
	FR 1.2 Acoustic comfort	x < dBA 30	Min	12.5
	FR 1.3 Accessible built environment for the elderly	Accessibility degree: 100%	Max	12.5
	FR 1.4 Adequate lighting	Δ700 lux = 0	Min	12.5
	FR 1.5 Green built environment	Leisure area m^2/person	Max	12.5
FR2: Unobtrusive building u.	FR 2.1 Minimize on-site works	Hours/ m^2	Min	12.5
	FR 2.2 Automated tools and Robotic devices	Automation degree = 100%	Max	12.5
	FR 2.3 Open building, flexibility	Application degree = 100%	Max	12.5
		SUM	Max	100

The quantitative research gap could be measured in a 0–100 scale. An Ideal Solution will formulate the objective. The ideal solution reaches 100 percent. For that purpose, the attributes must be assessed according to some indicators (Table 3.2). Again, these indicators can be changed, extended, or adapted depending on each assessment.

There are some indicators that need to be close to a certain value. For instance, in FR11 thermal comfort, there are several known indicators such as air speed, relative humidity, and natural ventilation. But for the assessment of these preliminary stages, only temperature will be considered as a main indicator. Therefore, a temperature close to 21°C (ΔT 21°C) will be taken as an indicator of a comfortable temperature. In FR12 acoustic comfort, there are also many other parameters to consider. FR 1.4 faces a similar situation as the previous attribute. It is known that lighting depends on the needs of the elderly at a particular time. But we will consider at least the minimum lux quantity (700 lux) for a safe situation.

There are some other indicators that need to be below or above a certain value. For instance, that is the case of FR 1.2, acoustic comfort. In this case, there exists several other indicators such as background noise, impact noise, etc., that can define acoustic comfort. In these early stages of assessment, only aerial noise in interiors of buildings will be considered. This noise should not exceed 30dB (x < dBA 30).

Some indicators have been chosen according to a percentage level. In FR 1.3, the percentage refers to the amount of accessible area for an elderly person in a wheel chair to access a defined built environment. In FR 2.2, the percentage refers to the degree of automation of the works carried out on-site. In FR 2.3, the percentage refers to the architectural infill elements that can be easily movable within a day.

Finally, there are indicators that are optimal in minimal or maximal values. That is the case of FR 1.5, green built environment. It has been considered that the greener the leisure area is, the better the elderly can enjoy. On the other hand, in FR2.1, it has been considered that the shorter the time used for upgrading each square meter of building, the better.

In this section, a list of attributes has been presented as a reference for future assessments of early strategies for BeuAAL. For a more detailed and accurate assessment, an MCDM should be applied.

3.5 Proposed Subsystems of BeuAAL with Automated and Robotic Devices

In Sections 3.2, 3.3, and 3.4, the main BeuAAL guidelines were outlined: First, the parameters for comfortable AAL built environment (Section 3.2) were set. Then, the parameters for an unobtrusive BeuAAL through automation and robotics (Section 3.3) were outlined. Finally, an assessment method for BeuAAL combining previous parameters was explained. Therefore, we can subtract a general scheme on how the BeuAAL divides into several subsystems. Except for the modular houses, every building has a different geometry, shape, and layout. Therefore, when approaching a rapid renovation process with prefabricated elements, we must consider that the prefabricated modules need to be bespoke or at least customized for each case. The customization does not matter only on the manufacturing process. The measurement, design, and installation processes are also very relevant. The product that will be installed onto the existing building must be carefully designed while considering these issues. Furthermore, the refurbishment protocols must be based on these criteria so that every element accurately fits into the space.

There have been research approaches for rapid building renovation and creation of totally bespoke building elements [135]. In this case, there is first an accurate measurement of the building. After that, the design of the drywall is adjusted to the measurement using CAD. With this design, the aluminum studs and plaster boards are cut accurately off-site. Finally, the elements are mounted on-site without making too much noise. In this case, the element was a common drywall. But since the accuracy gained was optimal, it could be used with modules with higher degrees of prefabrication, and probably with inner services.

3.5.1 Subsystem 1: Definition of the Upgrading Product, Element, or Module That Will Be Manufactured and Installed by Robots

In building construction, we find three main strategies for applying robotics:

- Configuring a product directly thanks to 3D printing devices.
- On-site assembly of small units or elements, such as bricks. In this case, there is a small degree of prefabrication. Subsequently, a high on-site robotic performance must be carried out, the robot must accomplish more tasks on-site.

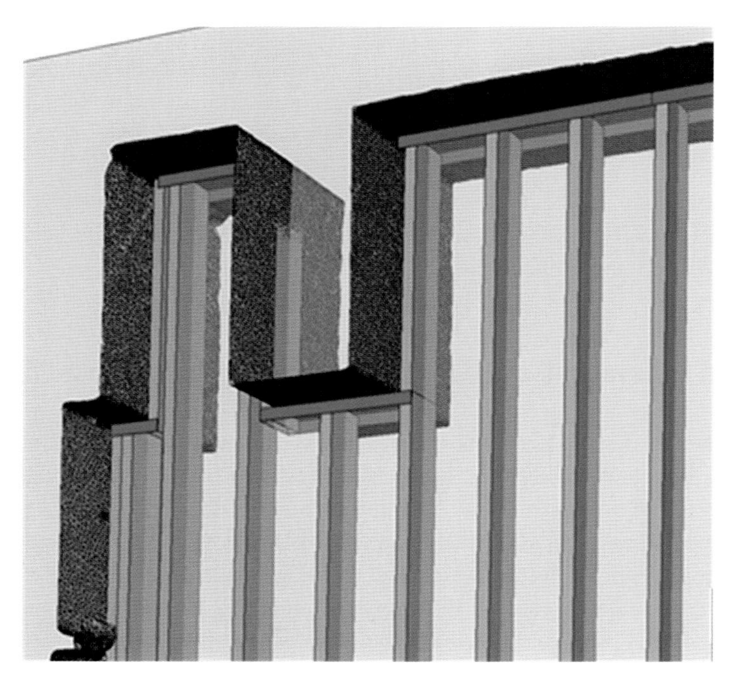

Figure 3.12 Accurate measurement of the existing building and bespoke manufacturing of the drywall studs by Prof. Dr. Ishida [135].
Source: Kogakuin University

- On-site assembly of prefabricated modules with a high-degree of prefabrication. In this case, the robotic performance is less complex than in the previous case.

When considering building upgrading for the elderly, these strategies need to be adjusted. The requirements are tighter. It must be considered, that in our case the performing scenario is not a workshop or a controlled environment, and not even a regular construction site. Which strategies are more accessible for building renovation? There are several factors that constrain the selection of one or other strategies:

- Operability in inner or outer existing built environments. It must be considered that the environments where the robots are working are livable. Therefore, hazardous and dirty situations must be avoided.
- Accuracy. Not only for the finishing, but specifically also for the services that must be installed with high precision.
- Executing speed. As stated in Section 3.3, the works must be unobtrusive to allow for minimal time.
- Logistics. Avoid bulky elements. For the internal parts of the building, 3D modules might be avoided in favor of 2D modules.
- Adaptability of the standard concept. Greater adaptability of the material, element or module and more flexible implementation on any kind of building type yields better results.

The level of standardization of the product takes a special role in the mass customization process. The adaptability degree must be foreseen.

3.5.2 Subsystem 2: Measurement and Data Acquisition of the Existing Building

Before attempting a building renovation process with robots, we must ensure that the accurate geometry of the building and the coordinates of every critical point are known. It must be clearly stated that the accurate data acquisition's main purposes are:

- Geometrical disposition of the existing building's elements in order to fit perfectly the upgrading element or module. The accurate measurement should provide bespoke items and avoid readjustment on-site.
- Accurate diagnosis of existing buildings' physical state. We must make sure that the support of the building is strong enough to host the new devices being inserted. Besides, issues related to heat transmission and insulation must be defined, especially if the renovation process deals with thermal improvement.
- Adequate robot path planning and task accomplishment. The robot needs to know beforehand where to perform the works.

If these premises are accomplished, the elements and the prefabricated module could fit correctly to the desired location without disturbing the stability of the building.

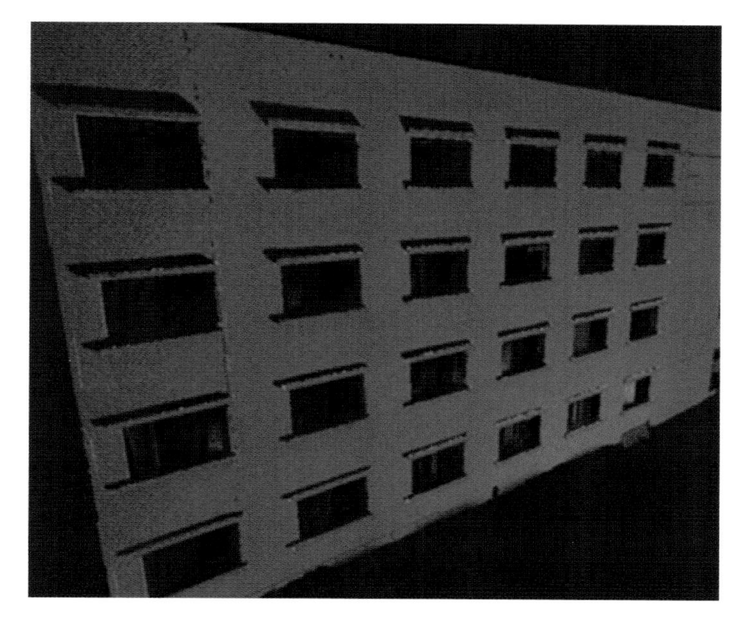

Figure 3.13 Point cloud of a facade.
Source: K. Iturralde

Focusing on the geometry of the building, the measurement of the existing built environment can be carried out using several devices:

- Digital tachometer or "Total station." This device measures the coordinates of the desired points. In other words, only the necessary points are acquired.
- Lidar or 3D LASER Scanning. With this laser tool, millions of points (point clouds) of the surrounding built environment can be collected in a few hours. These devices do not discriminate the collected points as in the previous case.
- Photogrammetry. In this case, the reconstruction of the building elements is made by reconstructed digital images.

The accuracy of the geometry acquired is higher with the digital tachometer than with the photogrammetric devices. Besides, in the case of the point clouds, the acquisition of these points requires an engineering process of transformation into a CAD or BIM model. Currently, considerable research has been developed on the automated generation of solid surfaces in CAD or BIM systems [136].

3.5.3 Subsystem 3: Disassembly or Removal of Unnecessary Elements in the Existing Buildings

During the renovation process, it is necessary to partially demolish some elements of the building. Among the building renovation tasks, this is one that is more problematic for automating. The biggest issues are:

- The current state of the built element is partially uncertain. With the current technology, it is difficult to have a completely accurate diagnosis of the building element that needs to be removed.
- The condition of the building can be damaged and some small or big elements can collapse. The robot must be programmed and controlled to these unforeseen situations. All the *physicalities* that the robot must accomplish must be foreseen.
- If the robot is performing outdoors, severe weather is a problem for the robot, it might disrupt the task of the robot or even damage it in some cases.

If the building elements can be easily disassembled instead of being removed, the process is less complex. Some robots that can perform this task have already developed [137]. This is definitely an interesting approach and more steps should be taken in order to achieve less risky and less dirty situations in building refurbishment.

3.5.4 Subsystem 4: Rapid Redesign processes using CAD, BIM, or Computational Design software

In Subsystem 1 it is explained how the building element or module that the robot must manufacture and/or install must be clearly defined. However, in building renovation, these elements or modules need to be adapted to each particular case. This adaptation is time-consuming if it is done manually with a software without a parametric tool.

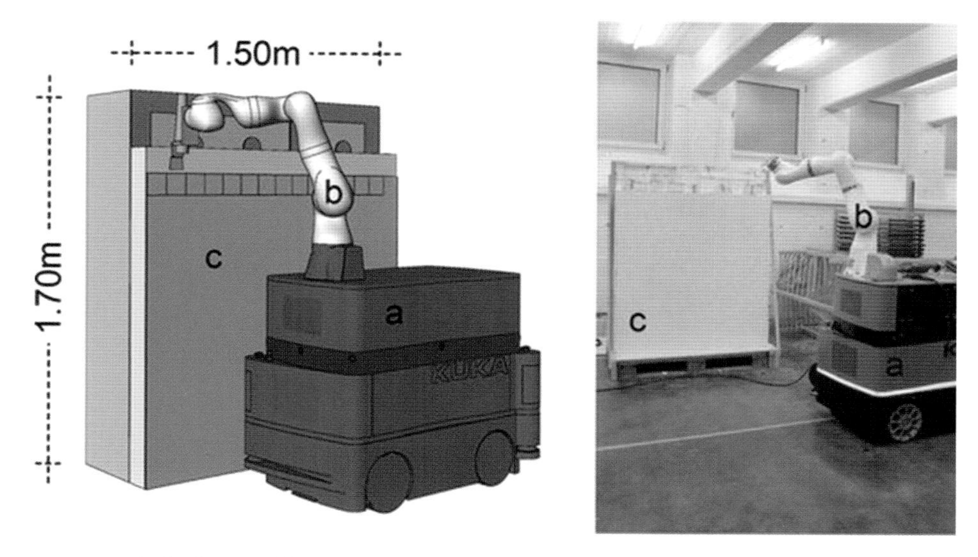

Figure 3.14 Robotic demolition of External Insulation Finishing System [137].
Source: Springer Nature

In the case of modules to be added onto existing facades, there are already several research projects that have developed specific parametric software tools. Besides, in the case of a prefabricated module, this adaptation must account for the intrinsic characteristics of each manufacturer, such as the shape of profiles, maximum size of modules, etc.

3.5.5 Subsystem 5: Accurate Manufacturing Processes of Bespoke Modules

The manufacturing process must enable customization of the modules. The factory layout and the workstations must be prepared to produce a changeable and variable product.

There are some experiences in the conception and implementation of customized products with robots. Two projects funded by the European Commission are developing techniques for the customization of timber prefab elements (SME robotics [140] and BERTIM [138] [139]). In all cases, the goal is to achieve efficient manufacturing processes.

3.5.6 Subsystem 7: Robotic Installation or On-Site Upgrading Process

The robots in building refurbishment need to foresee several constraints that are not necessary in the erection of new buildings. The biggest constraint is that the robot needs to adapt its path and performance to the building, which, as said before, is uncertain to a certain degree. Besides, the safety measures must be highly developed so as to be nonhazardous to

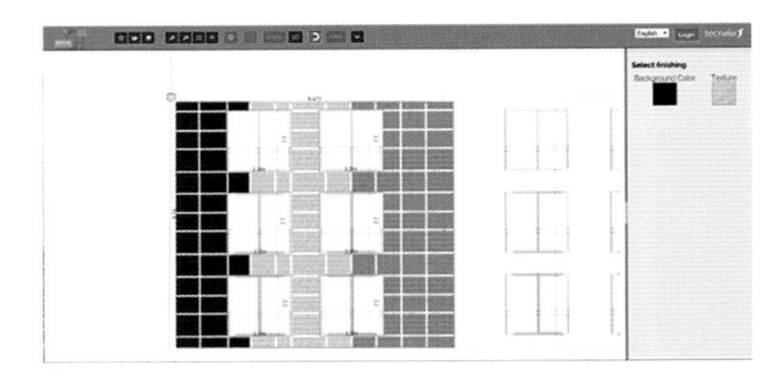

Figure 3.15 RenoBIM in the BERTIM project: 3D configurator based on the real BIM model of the building.
Source: BERTIM

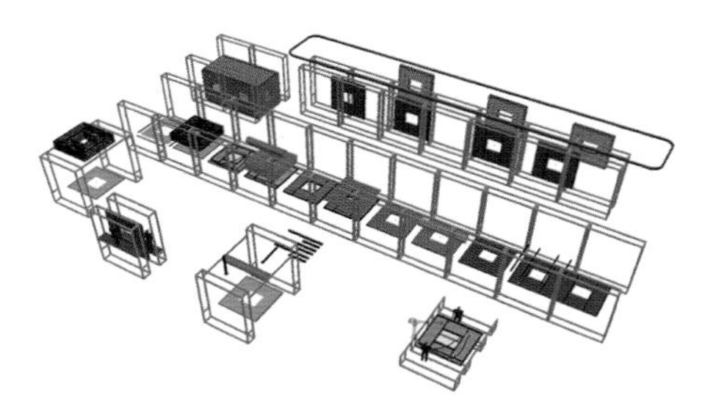

Figure 3.16 BERTIM Adaptable workstations for a customized manufacturing process [138] [139].
Source: K. Iturralde, BERTIM

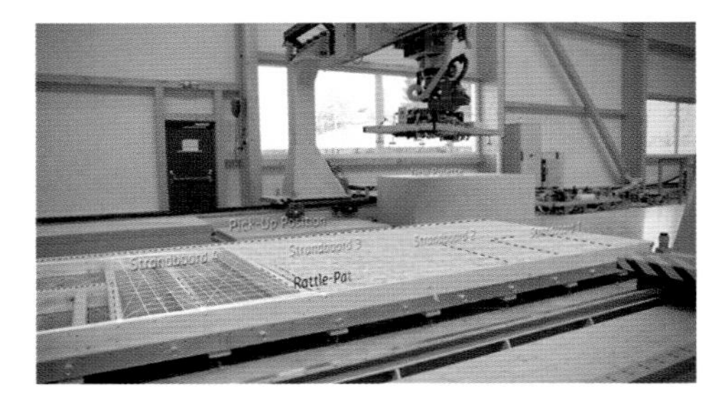

Figure 3.17 Robotic workstation for the manufacturing of prefab timber modules in SME robotics project [140].
Source: SME robotics

the inhabitants and users of the building. Regarding the difficulty of tasks, it can be mentioned that there are two degrees of complexity based on the workspace of the robot:

- 2D surfaces such as facades, walls, or floors. Here, it can be stated that the robot is working in a planar area.
- 3D environments, such as interiors of buildings. In this case, the robot must allocate itself and perform the works in a more complex environment.

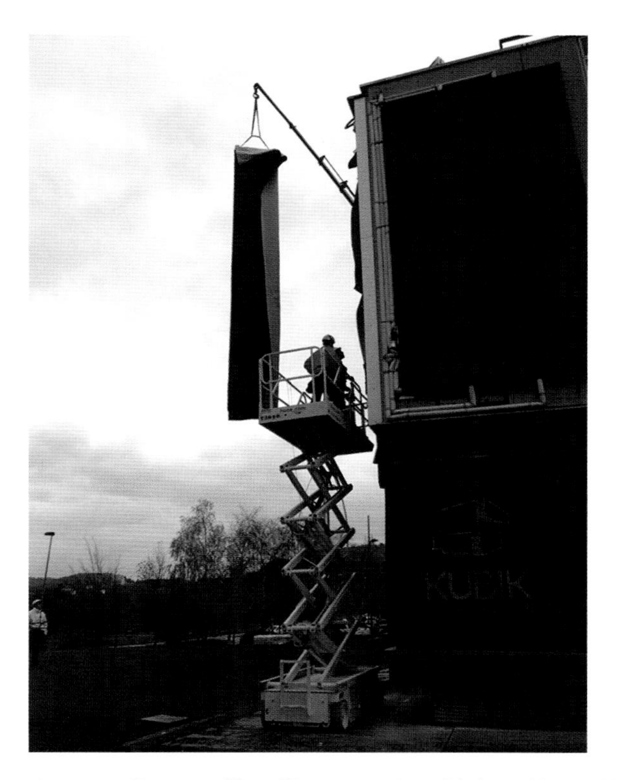

Figure 3.18 Process of installing external prefabricated layers [138] [139] with undedicated devices in the BERTIM process.
Source: BERTIM

In both cases, the robot body, the Degrees of Freedom (DOF) and the controlling system need to meet the requirements defined by each environment. Already, there are ongoing research projects that are dealing with this.

For that purpose, as mentioned before, the latest research projects have been developing prefabricated solutions and modules that include services, energy collection devices, insulation, and finishing material. This facilitates a rapid installation process and avoids rework tasks. However, the installation process of these modules could be more automated. We can define three main degrees of automation in the installation of prefabricated elements onto building envelopes:

- Lowest degree: there is no use of dedicated devices. The cranes and support platforms are conventional.
- Intermediate degree: the installation devices are specifically designed for lifting and placing the prefabricated modules.
- Robotic installation: a robot can install the main connecting system and the module itself. These devices are currently being developed, such as the Hephaestus Project [141] (see Figure 3.19).

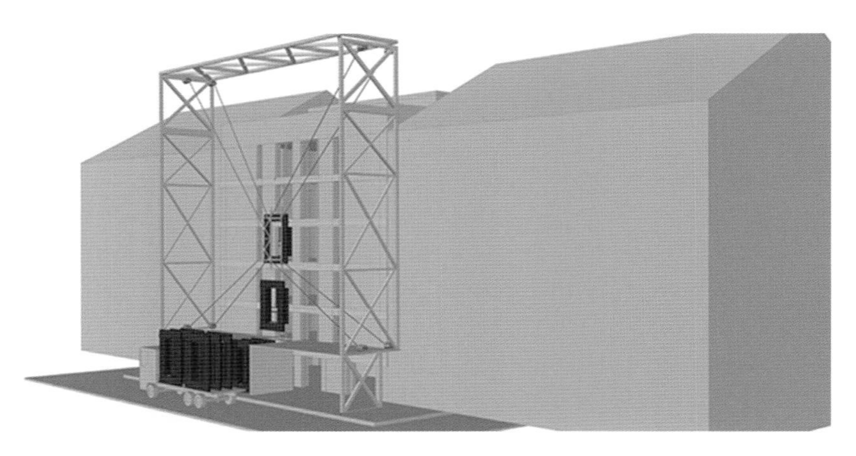

Figure 3.19 Robotic installation process using a cable driven robot within the Hephaestus Project [141]. European Union's Horizon 2020 research and innovation program under grant agreement No 732513.
Source: K. Iturralde

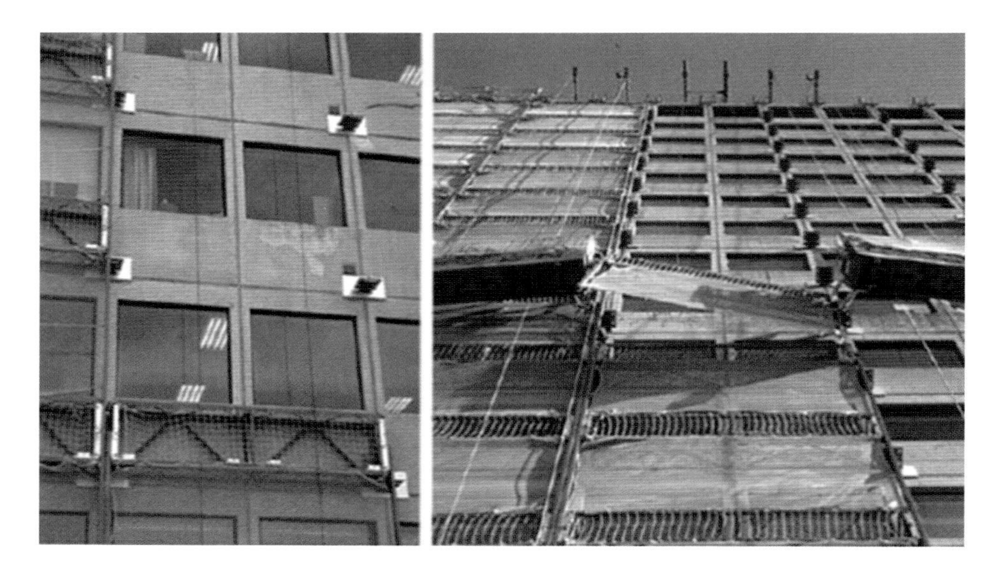

Figure 3.20 OMM building renovation in Osaka (Japan) using dedicated devices for installation in 1989.
Source: YKK AP

A very interesting example of adding a new layer on the envelope of the building was achieved at the OMM building in Osaka, Japan. Here, the whole process was carried out without any need of evacuating all the users. The project was based on the prefabricated curtain wall module. The measurement, adjustment and placement of the connectors had a primordial relevance for a fast installation process (Figure 3.20).

3.6 Adaptable Building Concepts

Several research projects and developments have been carried out in the last years with the aim of developing an adaptable building. The needs of existing society are changing and therefore built stock should shift toward solutions that are more adequate to these requirements. In this chapter, two projects will be explained.

3.6.1 Project A2L-Mobilius

The phenomenon of urbanization has reached an unprecedented level. According to a recent UN report, around 55 percent of the global population is considered to be living in urban areas, and the number is expected to rise to 68 percent by 2050 [142]. A number of megacities emerged during the process of rapid urbanization. Among these, Cairo, the capital of Egypt, is arguably the largest metropolis in Africa, and one of the largest in the world. More than two-thirds of Greater Cairo Region's metropolitan residents live in informal urban settlements, and the number is set to increase continuously, which creates serious issues such as overcrowding, land shortage, high unemployment, inadequate infrastructure, lack of basic services, and environmental pressure [143]. Therefore, the situation would be even more problematic if no innovative solutions are implemented in the near future. The project A2L-Mobilius aims to explore an integrated building system to tackle the aforementioned issues as well as to revitalize the local communities in Cairo's informal settlements. Through an investigation of informal settlements in Cairo, an Affordable and Adaptable Building System (A^2BS) is proposed. Decentralized Processing Units (DPUs) tailored to the building system are presented to enhance three main aspects of life: working, energy and mobility. Furthermore, a simulation of a regenerated house based on a selected case study building is demonstrated, which integrates A^2BS and various DPUs. Last, but not least, a proper business strategy for the future prosperity of the local communities is discussed based on Decentralized Industrial Village (DIV) concept [144].

Methodology

The project uses the V-Model diagram (see Figure 3.21) the methodology, which is derived from Software Engineering (SE). This method allows the project to be divided into smaller work packages, which can be addressed by one design module or a sum of modules [145].

Collaboration with the local stakeholders is crucial to the success of this project. Therefore, it is important to ensure the participation and feedback from stakeholders throughout the project. Based on the requirements of engineering [146], the project team developed a methodology that considers repetitive optimization loops to constantly monitor and optimize the stakeholder analysis and requirements analysis throughout the project. The purpose of the requirements analysis, together with a technological feasibility study, is to identify functions that can be interpreted into design elements, and to establish a suitable common structure for the project (see Figure 3.22).

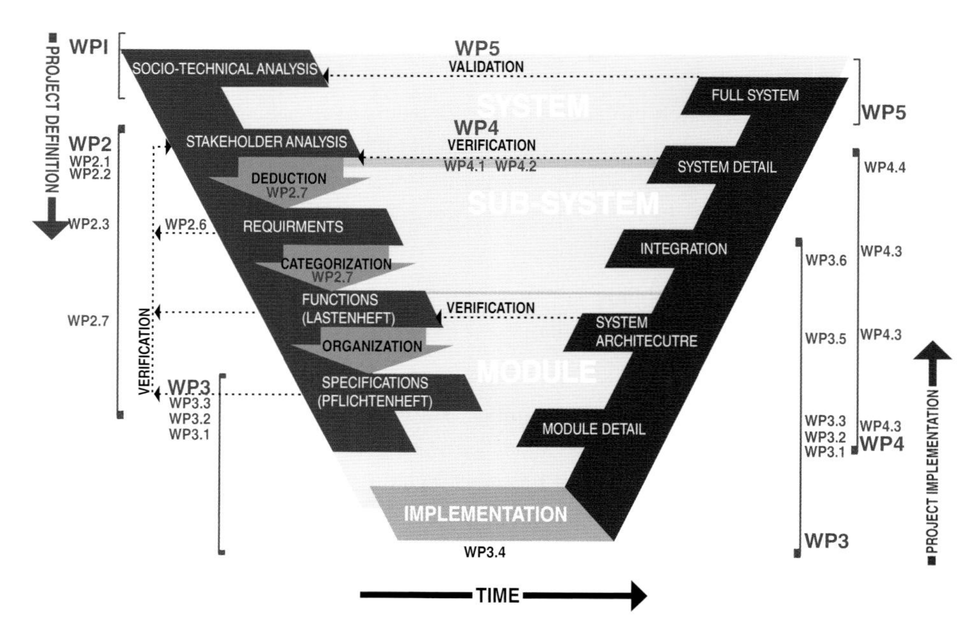

Figure 3.21 V-Model for the A2L-Mobilius project [144].
Source: C. Follini and R. Hu

Affordable and Adaptable Building System

Based on the aforementioned analyses, the project team proposed A²BS, which is a flexible and affordable building system composed of prefabricated elements. The system, specially designed to fit the informal environment, can adapt over time to local dwellers' needs. The objective of the system is to incrementally replace the informal housing and thus "formalize" the built environment. The design of A²BS is based on Open Building principles [129], [147], which include three subsystems: the modular structural subsystem, the building envelope subsystem, and the service infill subsystem (see Figure 3.23).

A modular concrete structural system is developed, which has the potential to both vertically and horizontally expand. This proposed structural system, which includes the concrete elements and the connecting beams in between, can easily be prefabricated either on site or off in a low-tech manner by untrained workers. As shown on the right side of the diagrams in Figure 3.24, the connecting beams have two dimensions: 2 m and 3.5 m in length, which comply with Cairo's common housing standards (see Figure 3.24).

The system has indicated substantial potential to mitigate the issues of rapid urbanization and urban poverty because the building can be erected and extended over time to ease the financial burden and to meet the needs of increasing population. Residents can choose the materials they prefer (bricks, wood, aluminum panels, concrete, etc.) to fill up the reserved spaces. Furthermore, the local dwellers are encouraged to participate in

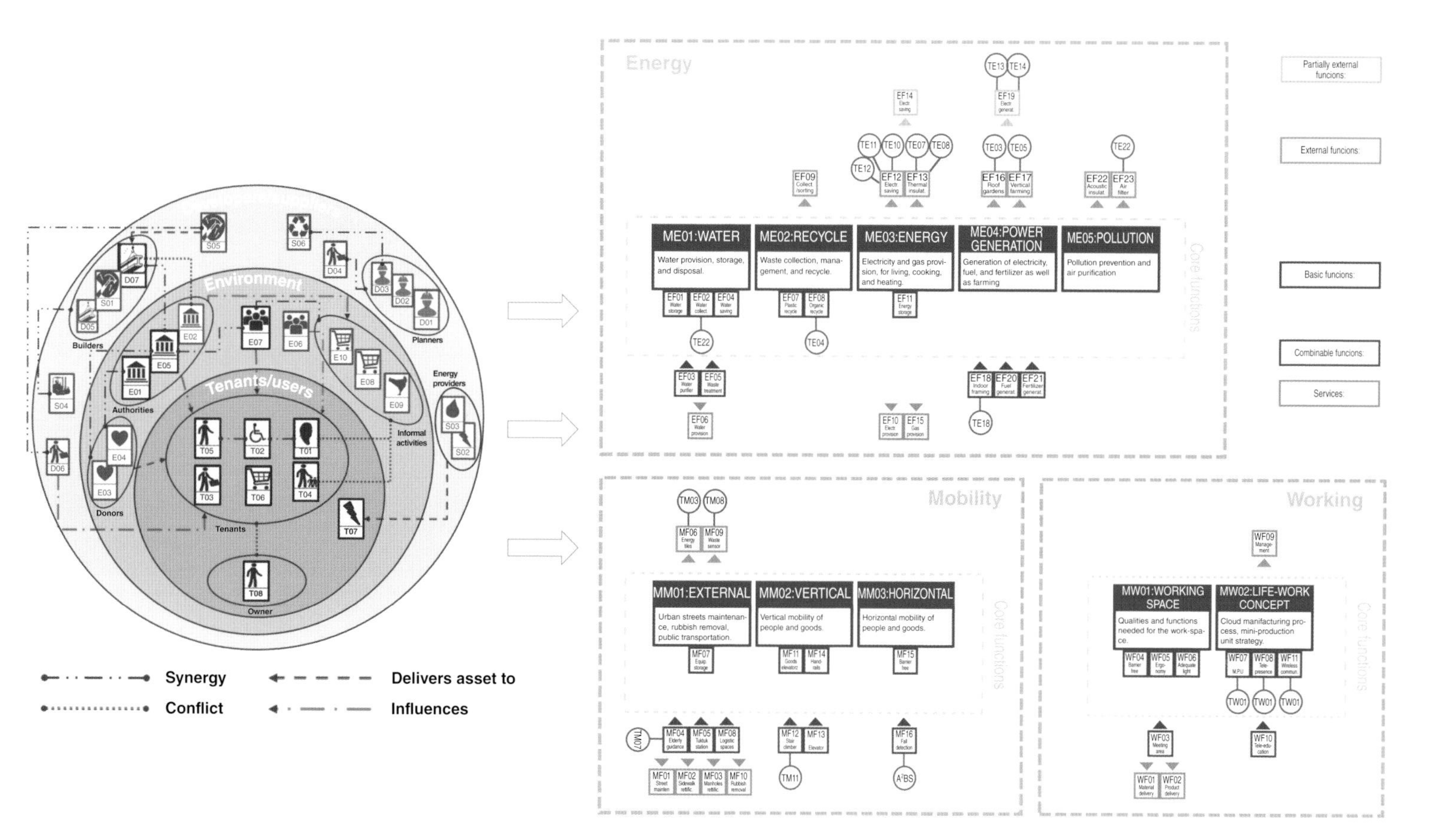

Figure 3.22 The results of stakeholder analysis (left) and requirements analysis (right) [144].
Source: C. Follini and R. Hu

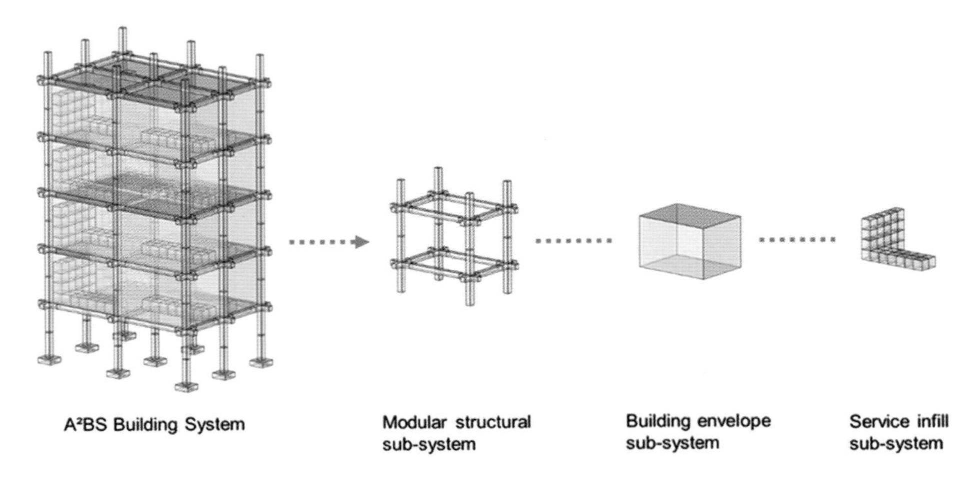

Figure 3.23 Schematic diagram of A²BS Building System [144].
Source: R. Hu

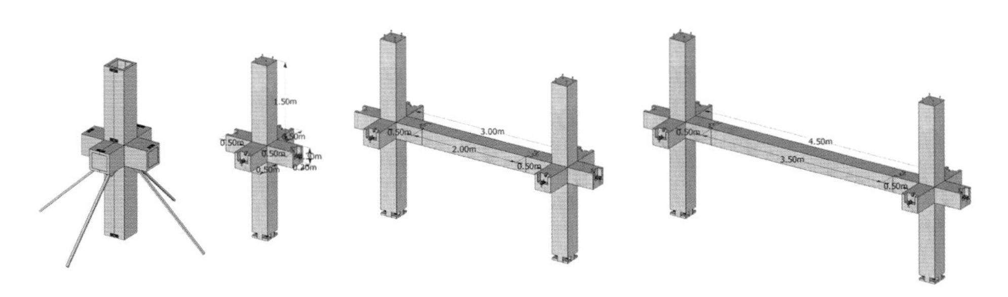

Figure 3.24 Modular concrete structural system [144].
Source: R. Hu

the construction and extension process of their own homes, as the building system is designed in a user-friendly and low-tech manner. In the future, when further living space is demanded as the residents' financial status improves or the number of the family members grows, the structure itself can also be vertically and horizontally extended with newly built structural elements. Figure 3.25 represents a scenario of a 30-year development of a building based on A²BS system.

Decentralized Processing Unit (DPU)

DPU represents a prefabricated, self-sustaining, interchangeable, and standardized system. It easily integrates a series of technological equipment needed for a household. Furthermore, it allows for a systematic upgrade of the informal settlements. The DPUs are tailor-made for the A²BS and are developed as decentralized units, which work together as one. This design decision allows for high variability in function, translating

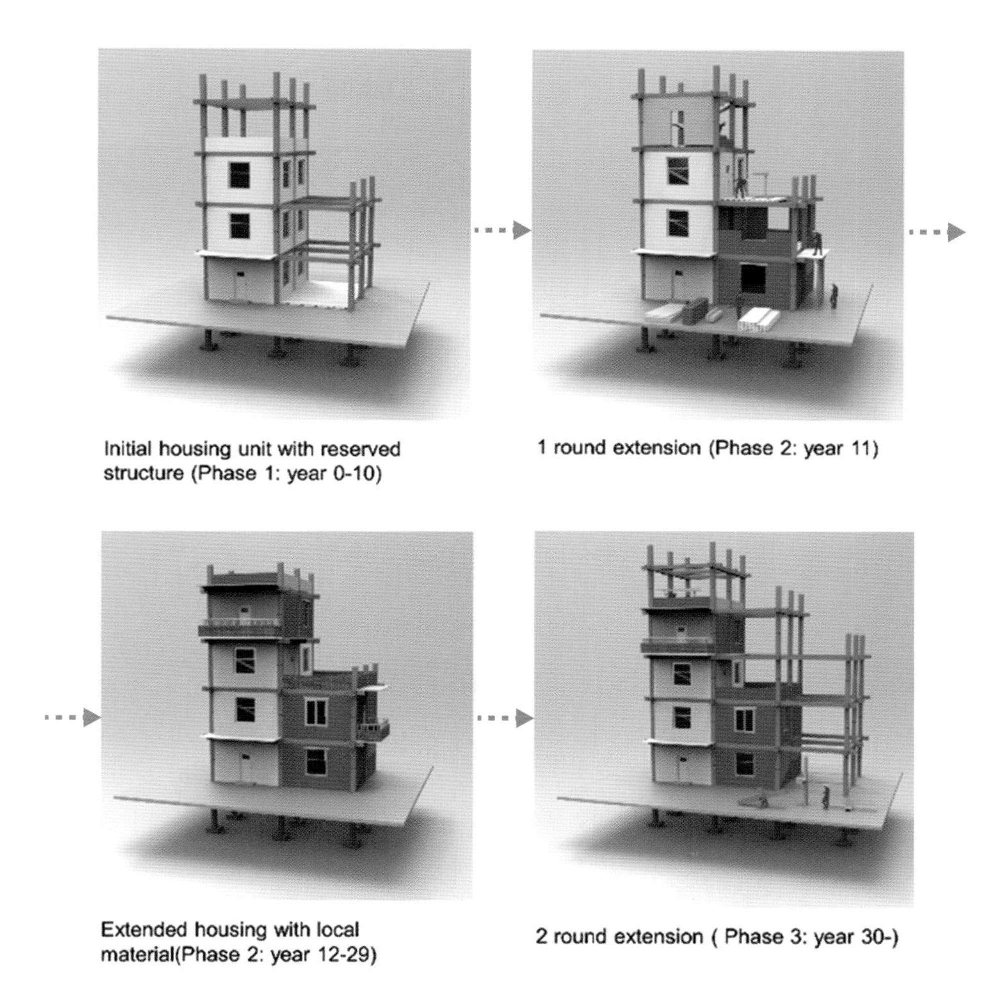

Figure 3.25 Thirty-year expansion scenario of A²BS Building System [144].
Source: R. Hu

into affordability and adaptability. A DPU comprises three subsystems: one for energy collection, provision, wise-use, and production; another for mobility improvement; and lastly one for life-work balance. The last one may serve as a mini production unit or mini home office (see Figure 3.26). Due to the specially made design, the DPU will be integrated easily into the modular building system (i.e., A²BS), which is fully reusable, further increasing affordability.

Decentralized Industrial Village

The Decentralized Industrial Village (DIV) concept describes a village, in which decentralized manufacturing workshops produce a series of components. The self-production will streamline the process, while preserving the existing urban context and profit of local

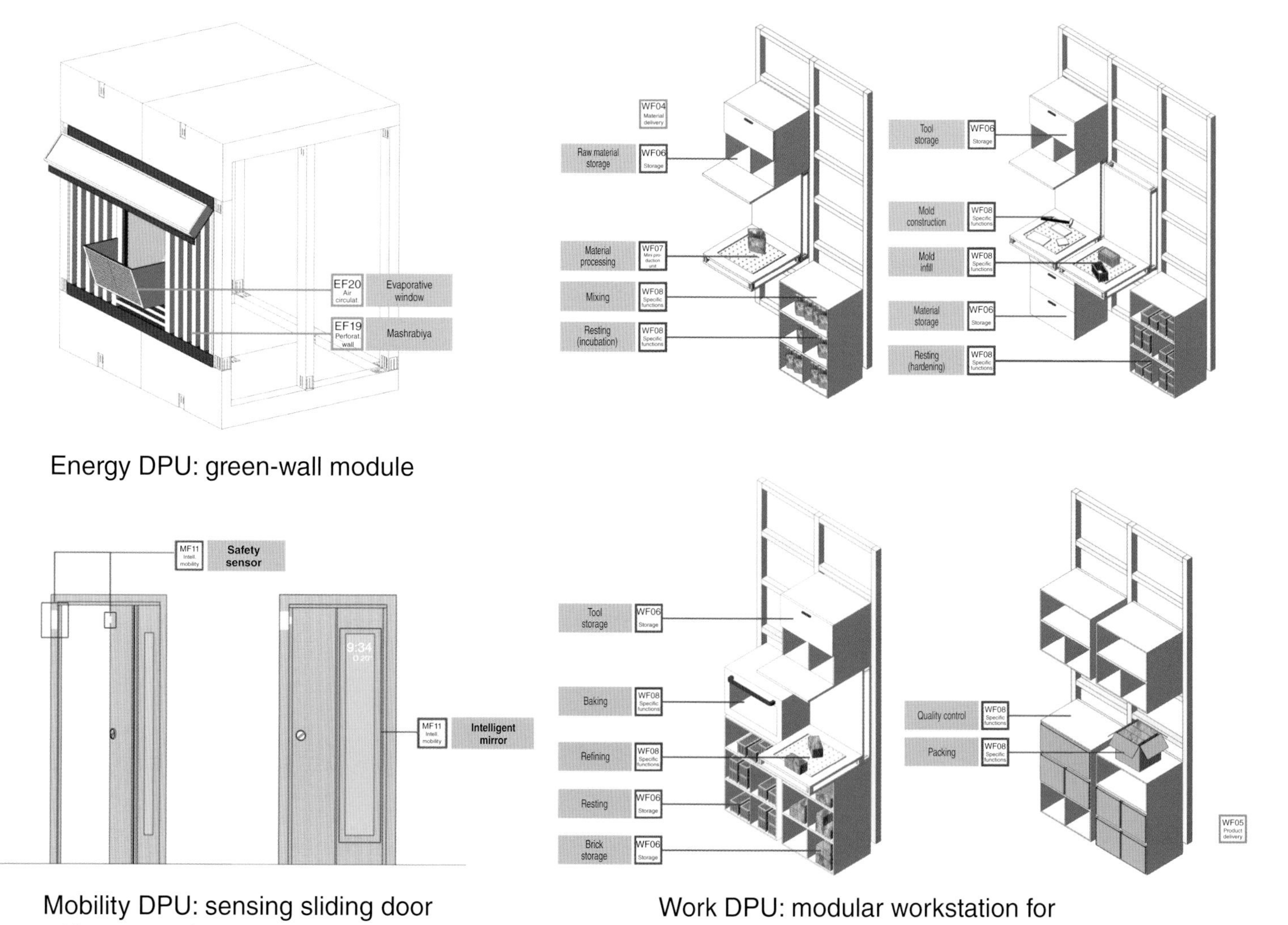

Figure 3.26 Three examples of DPUs which can be embedded A^2BS [148].
Source: C. Follini and R. Hu

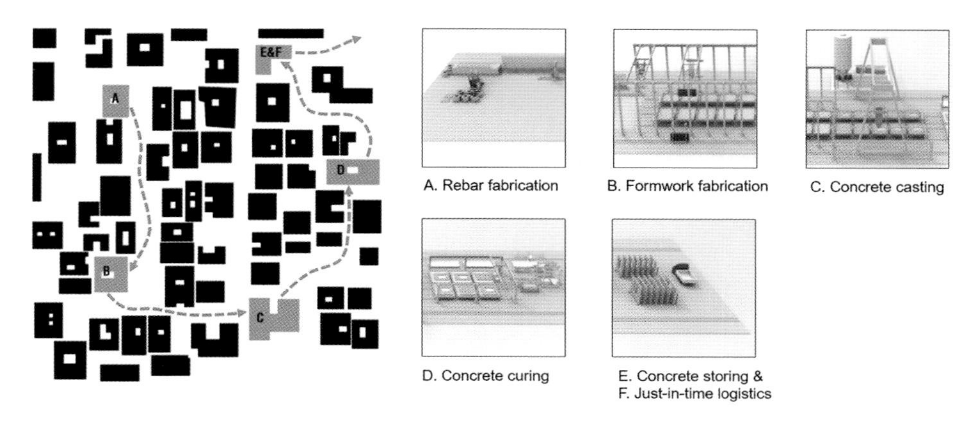

Figure 3.27 Exemplary business model in the Decentralized Industrial Village [144]. Source: R. Hu

business. The exploitation of a profitable business model, i.e. DIV, is a feasible method to reduce the unemployment rate for the local people and therefore revitalizing the informal settlements. To promote this innovative model, it is proposed to transform part of Cairo into DIV. There are many possibilities to manufacture innovatively within the DIV, e.g., to prefabricate the aforementioned modular building components. These then can be utilized in the regeneration of the local community. The procedures include rebar fabrication, formwork fabrication, concrete casting, curing, storing, and transport, which can be allocated to different households nearby (see Figure 3.27).

Integration and Simulation

In the Sakiat Mekki area of Giza District in Cairo, there is a four-story housing unit with a 45 m^2 apartment on each floor. This case study demonstrates the potential application of the A^2BS system and the DPUs. The ground floor is an active mechanical workshop. The first floor is owned by a single woman living and working alone at home. The second floor houses a family of four, but only during the summer. The third floor is unoccupied. The roof is used by all residents as a common space for various types of gatherings. Finally, the stairs are used as extra space for washing, cooking, and storage. These stairs have no handrails and the risers have height differences. Despite the apparent liveability of the building, there are various issues including lack of garbage cans, noise from workshops in the ground floor, lack of ventilation, lack of handrails, risers of different heights, sanitation issues, and space shortage [148]. Moreover, horizontal extension is not possible. Due to the current state of the case study, it is proposed to simulate a complete upgrade by integration of the A2BS system and a series of DPUs (see Figure 3.28 and Table 3.3). The only permanent resident is the single woman on the first floor, so the relocation process during construction would be smooth and easy. The construction process would be rapid due to the flexible and modular building system.

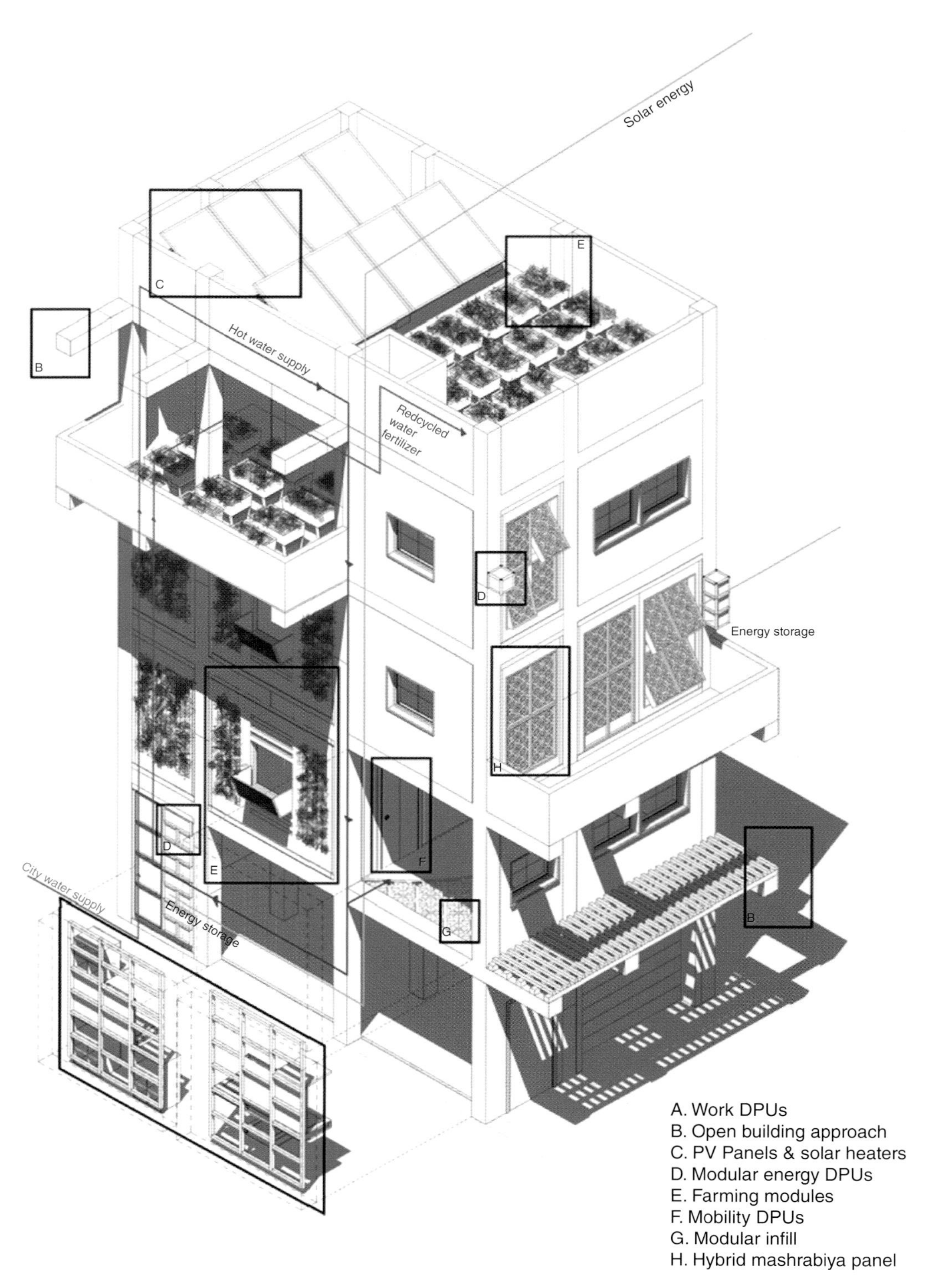

Figure 3.28 A simulation of regeneration based on the case study building village [144]. Source: C. Follini and R. Hu

Table 3.3 Details of Technologies Integrated into the Case Study Building

A. Work DPUs	The modular working station has been tailored to the case study to develop the business model [149]. The station proposed contains four main steps of production, and the different workstations can be distributed in the settlements. The workstations will resemble equipped walls to save space to allow for direct mounting on the A^2BS system.
B. Open Building Concept	The concept of Open Building (OB), also known as Support/Infill (S/I), is now representing one of the most flexible construction principles. The building has been designed in different levels: support structures, infill system, fit-out, and appliances. These have been repurposed to harness the benefits of state-of-the-art industrial production, emerging information and digital technologies, improved logistics, and changing social values and market structures.
C. PV Panels and Solar Heaters	The solar panel is a broadly known technology for collecting solar energy. Composed of small silicon cells, they convert solar energy into either electricity or heat. Nowadays at a relatively reasonable price, the project will utilize solar panels for both purposes: some will provide additional electricity that will be stored in the DPU cluster on the ground floor; some will heat the water received from the city supply before distribution to the different apartments.
D. Modular Energy DPUs	The energy subsystem provides reliability and responsiveness to the needs of the community related to collection, provision, wise-use and eventual production of different kinds of primary resources such as electricity, gas, and water. The functions of the energy subsystem have been sorted into five main clusters, based on their scope: water, recycle, electricity, power generation, and ventilation. The function clusters try to address the most relevant issues related to energy consumption, collection, and saving. The DPU physical modules that accommodate the different technologies for this purpose have different shapes and dimensions. Figure 3.28 represents one example, the "box" modules, which are to be installed individually or in clusters and then attached to the A^2BS structure. The joints will make it feasible to install and detach easily the modules, increasing the flexibility of the system.
E. Farming Modules	The project considers the use of rooftop aeroponic technology, which refers to a technology allowing plants to grow without soil or another aggregate media. Plants are irrigated periodically with fresh air, water, and nutrients 24 hours per day. Meanwhile, vertical farming is applied to the installation of green walls on building façades. Green walls are usually composed of a frame that hosts soil to grow climbing plants. There are many advantages of vertical farming, such as insulation, evaporative cooling, temperature reduction, and space saving [150].
F. Mobility DPUs	Firstly, one approach proposed for the mobility subsystem is a gradual modification of the interior in the form of Mobility DPUs, aiming to "infect" the environment and provide gradual upgrades. Thus, the stair and door modules with sensors have been elaborated to seamlessly integrate with the interior space. Secondly, exterior mobility is also considered concerning a typical instance of Egyptian small range mobility is the tuk-tuks, which are popular privately-owned vehicles that serve as public transportation. A similar concept is employed by the VOI electric motorcycle, developed by TUM Create [151]. Similar to a tuk-tuk, the vehicle can transport one passenger at a time. Moreover, it is equipped with an interchangeable capsule in the front, which hosts various pods. The functions vary from passenger transport to delivery of goods. This approach would be ideal because the local streets are often overcrowded with insufficient space for mobility.

Table 3.3 *(cont.)*

G. Modular Infill	The modular infill system is to be embedded as the "second layer" of the building, while the modular structure as the "first layer." It provides a framework that will accommodate different ranges of functional modules. The framework consists of the wall frame and floor module, where both are easily connected with and detached from the structure when replacement is needed. Basic electrical wiring and pipes will run through the framework, by internally adding a layer of plasterboard to provide a finished wall. The material of the wall frame can be locally sourced. The floor module is made of fire-resistant polystyrene material, enabling flexible installation of pipes and other services. The floorboards above the floor module can be easily removed, in order to gain access to the pipes and services.
H. Hybrid Mashrabiya Panel	Mashrabiya refers to a traditional architectural element especially applied in Islamic culture with both aesthetic and functional purposes. Its functions include, but are not limited to controlling light and air direction, reducing temperature, and providing privacy. Size, pattern, and distance from balusters determine the extent of employment of these functions. The proposed solution has a hybrid approach of using photovoltaic with traditional Mashrabiya. The photovoltaic film is attached to the frame carved with the traditional pattern. Different technologies are considered for the film, which is required to be transparent, in order not to block the view from the window. The electricity will be stored in the DPU clusters on the ground floor, serving the whole building [152].

Conclusion

In order to tackle the aforementioned issues of informal settlements in Cairo, this research explores an integrated approach to improve the living condition of local residents, thus revitalizing the local communities. By investigating the status quo and urgent needs of Cairo's informal settlements with a scientific methodology, an Affordable and Adaptable Building System (A^2BS) based on open building concepts is proposed, which can be easily prefabricated and assembled by unskilled workers. Meanwhile, Decentralized Processing Units (DPUs) customized to A^2BS are introduced to enhance three main aspects of life (working, energy, and mobility). In addition, a simulation of regenerated case study building is presented, which integrates A^2BS and various DPUs. Furthermore, a suitable business model for the local communities is identified based on the Decentralized Industrial Village (DIV) concept. The proposed system is favorable according to the local residents and stakeholders' feedback during site visits. The proposed system can be further adjusted according to the feedback (improved dimensions of the structural system, improved load distribution on the roof, optimized layout of the Decentralized Industrial Village, etc.). In conclusion, this research raises public awareness of the challenges and opportunities in Cairo's informal settlements, provides a valuable framework to researchers, architects and urban planners in the related fields, and takes a step forward to improve the living conditions of informal settlements in Cairo and worldwide [144].

3.6.2 Dynamic Vertical Urbanism

Like a sophisticated organism, a city has an essential characteristic which is the ability to constantly and flexibly transform throughout its lifecycle in response to economy shifts, demographic change, and environmental pressures. Nowadays, megacities in China are confronted with unprecedented challenges such as overcrowding, population aging, land shortage, traffic congestion, and environmental pressures during the process of uncontrollable urban sprawl. Therefore, to mitigate the aforementioned issues, a number of new developments entitled "Vertical City" have emerged. However, few of them represent one key feature of a city, which is the ability to grow and transform. Dynamic Vertical Urbanism features constant vertical urban transformation by applying the state-of-the-art construction technologies. Inspired by Hutong, a type of vernacular community in China commonly formed by traditional courtyard residences, this Vertical City concept has the ability to integrate five basic elements of a city [153]: vertical and horizontal circulation systems as its paths, a flexible building envelope as its edges, various mix-used building blocks as its districts, sky bridges and roof gardens as its nodes, and the complex itself as a landmark. More importantly, it can change its size, form and function with the help of technologies such as Robot-oriented Design [154], construction automation, Open Building principles [129], and Process Information Modelling [155] (see Figure 3.29).

Integrated with an on-site construction factory (OCF) on top of each tower, Dynamic Vertical Urbanism has the ability to responsively evolve in accordance with social, economic, and environmental shifts in a self-sufficient manner, meanwhile avoiding the risk of being homogeneous with surrounding buildings. A possible scenario for the

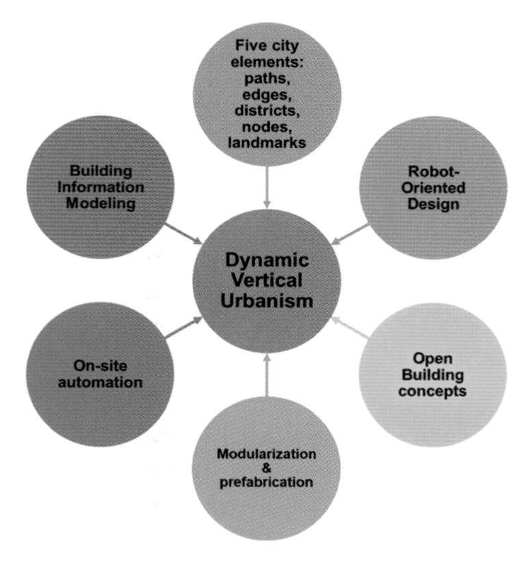

Figure 3.29 Six pillars in the novel Vertical City approach [156].
Source: R. Hu and W. Pan

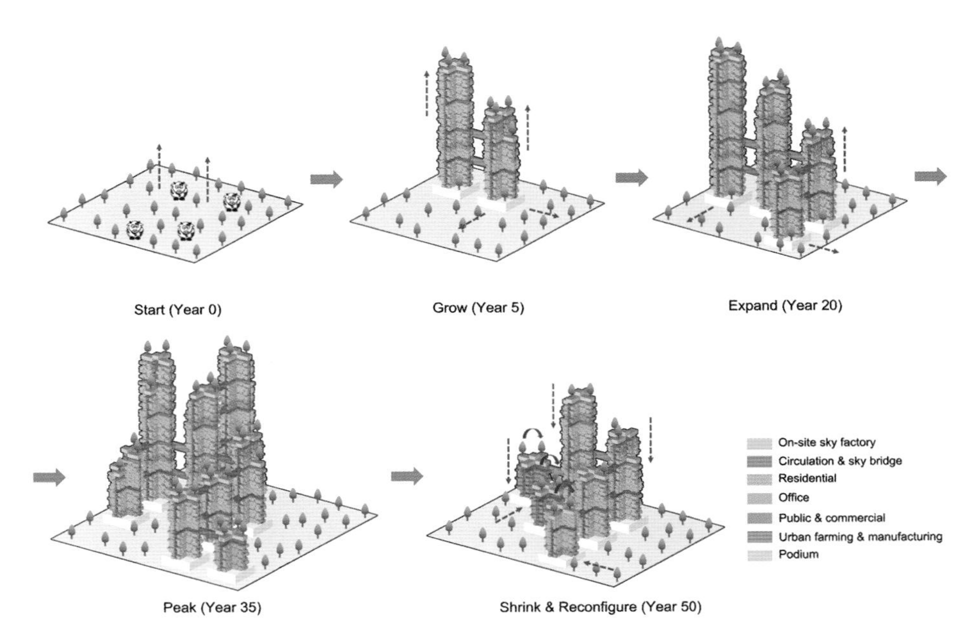

Figure 3.30 A typical scenario of a 50-year development of a Dynamic Vertical Urbanism complex [156]. Source: R. Hu and W. Pan

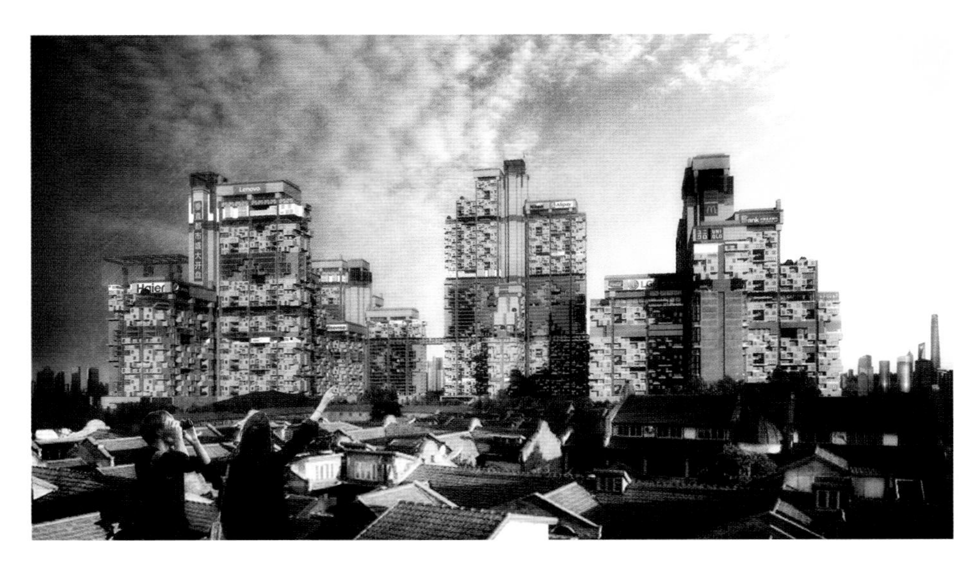

Figure 3.31 A typical scenario of a 50-year development of a Dynamic Vertical Urbanism complex [156]. Source: R. Hu and W. Pan

future development over the lifecycle of a building complex following Dynamic Vertical Urbanism principles is envisioned in Figure 3.30.

Eventually, the complex will perform as a series of interlinked components that collaborate together to form a sophisticated urban organism which provides various

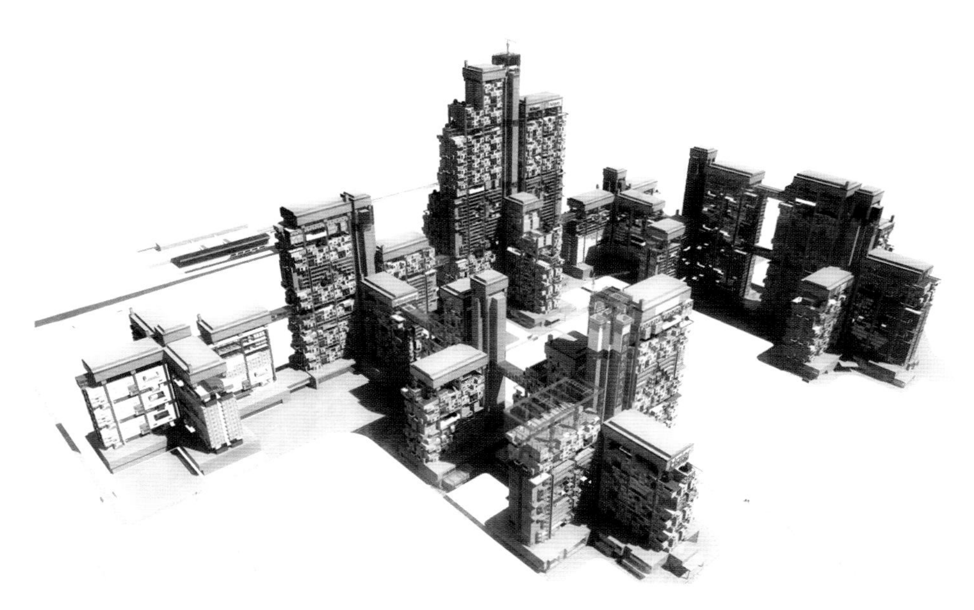

Figure 3.32 Aerial view of the proposed complex following Dynamic Vertical Urbanism principles [156]. Source: R. Hu and W. Pan

functions such as corporate, residential, commercial, academic, medical, legal, and infrastructural (see Figure 3.31 and Figure 3.32). In conclusion, this study provides researchers, architects and urban planners with a valuable framework for developing Vertical Cities, thus potentially triggering a paradigm shift in future urban transformation process in China and around the world [156].

4 Existing AAL Products

In this chapter, several technological, or to be more detailed, robotic solutions from different companies and developers will be presented. This allows an overview of the state of Ambient/Active Assisted Living (AAL), which can be categorized into home care (for independent living in old age), social interaction, health and wellness, interaction and learning, working, and mobility.

4.1 Home Care (Independent Living)

Here, an overview about robotics which are used in the home care field is given. In Table 4.1, a short overview about the robots introduced in this section is presented.

System Name: PaPeRo
Developer: NEC Corporation
PaPeRo is a "Personal Robot" best known for its recognizable appearance and facial recognition abilities (see Figure 4.1). PaPeRo, which stands for "**Pa**rtner-type-**Pe**rsonal-**Ro**bot" was developed as a personal assistant that could interact with people in everyday life situations. It is equipped with a variety of abilities for interaction. For example, if asked, "Is today a good day for a drive?," PaPeRo will autonomously connect to the internet, assess the weather forecast for the day, and provide a recommendation. It also has the ability to play games with people, provide music for a party, and imitate both in voice and movement. PaPeRo adapts to various personalities based on the types of interaction it receives (tone of voice, frequency of interaction, type of question asked, etc.) and develops a simulated mood based on the moods of the humans it interacts with. When not given any immediate tasks, PaPeRo roams around searching for faces and once one is found, will begin conversing with it.
Technology: PaPeRo's distinguishing "eyes" are in fact two cameras that allow for its visual awareness and facial recognition system. A pair of sensitive microphones allow the system to determine where, and from whom, human speech is coming from using its speech recognition system and PaPeRo will react accordingly. It is also equipped with an ultrasound system in order to detect obstacles. If an object is in its path, the exact location of the object will be detected and a route avoiding the object will be designed and employed. Source: www.nec.co.jp.

System Name: Mamoru-Kun
Developer: Center of IRT (CIRT), Tokyo University
Mamoru-Kun is an assistive robot for seniors (see Figure 4.1). The purpose of the robot is to remind users where they may have left often-misplaced items such as keys, glasses, or slippers. Reminders can be provided either verbally or the robot can physically point out the

Table 4.1 Overview about Robots Introduced in this Chapter

System Name	Developer
PaPeRo (Partner-type-Personal-Robot)	NEC Corporation
Mamoru-Kun	Center of IRT (CIRT), Tokyo University
Emiew 2 (Excellent Mobility and Interactive Existence as Workmate)	Hitachi
Home Assistant AR	Center of IRT (CIRT), Tokyo University
Twendy-One	Waseda University
My Spoon	Secom
Maron-1	Fujitsu
NetTansorWeb	Bandai and Evolution Robotics

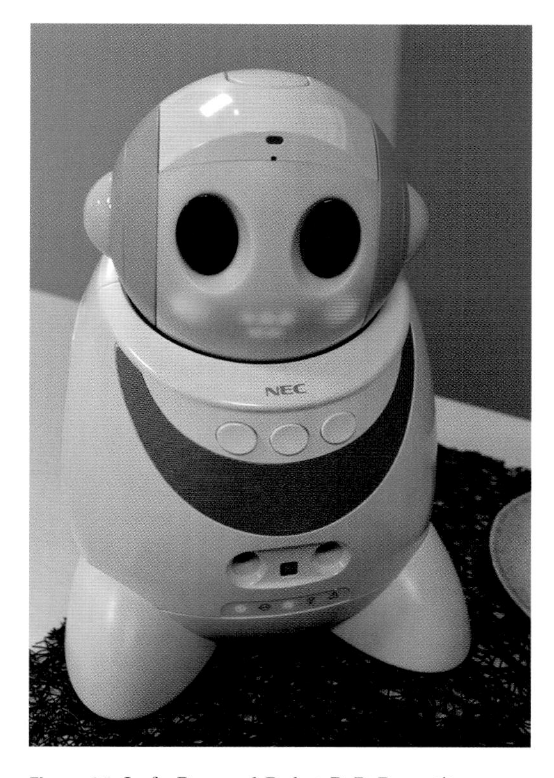

Figure 4.1 Left: Personal Robot PaPeRo petit.
Source: YOSHIKAZU TSUNO/AFP/Getty Images

location of the items. Alternatively, it can communicate with its older brother, the "Home Assistance Robot," and have it retrieve the desired items. Mamoru can also be programmed to provide everyday reminders such as taking one's medication.

Technology: Mamoru is primarily an "Object-Recognition-Robot," equipped with a wide-angle lens. It stands 40 cm tall and weighs 3.8 kg. It has four joints (two in the neck and one in each arm), a microphone, and speakers in order to communicate the location of lost items. In order for personal items to be identified and located, users must register their often-misplaced items in advance to create a sort of inventory for the robot. If the item is within the system's field of view, object recognition software is able to identify it and inform the user of its location. Source: www.irt.i.u-tokyo.ac.jp.

System Name: Emiew 2
Developer: Hitachi
The second iteration of Emiew (**E**xcellent **M**obility and **I**nteractive **E**xistence as **W**orkmate, see Figure 4.2) was developed by Hitachi. Emiew is a service robot with diverse communication abilities that could safely and comfortably coexist with humans while carrying out necessary services. Its communication is supported with a vocabulary of about 100 words. In order to achieve higher mobility speeds, Emiew was designed with two wheels as "feet" and can travel up to 6 km/h. At the time of development, the previous version of Emiew was the fastest moving service robot yet. With sensors on its head, waist, and near the base, Emiew is able to interact with users and follow various commands. Its speed and abilities make Emiew particularly useful in the office setting to assist in running various errands.
Technology: Emiew stands 80 cm tall and weighs just 13 kg, has a maximum speed of 6 km/h and an impressive acceleration of 4 m/s^2. A specially developed two-wheel mechanism allows Emiew to travel at a rate comparable to humans. An "active suspension" system consisting of a spring and an actuator gives Emiew agility and the ability to roll over small differences in floor levels and various office obstacles such as cables. Emiew is equipped with no fewer than

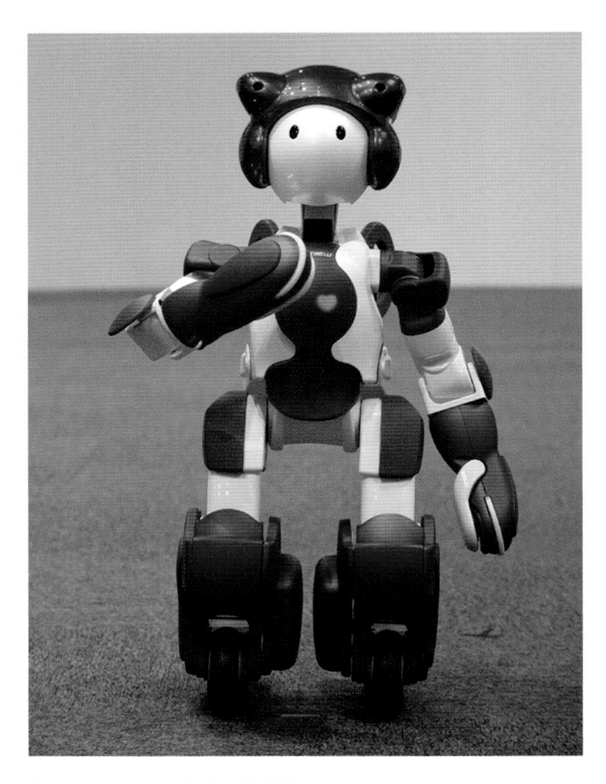

Figure 4.2 (a) Left: EMIEW3.
Source: TOSHIFUMI KITAMURA/AFP/Getty Images

14 microphones to allow for accurate voice detection including directionality. The robot is also equipped with noise-cancellation technology in order to filter out the noise created by the robot itself, and better focus on that of the users. A series of sensors allows the robot to acutely detect obstacles – either stationary or moving (e.g., people) – and efficiently navigate its way through them in order to quickly reach its destination. Source: www.engadget.com.

System Name: Home Assistant AR
Developer: Center of IRT (CIRT), Tokyo University
AR (shown in Figure 4.2) is a humanoid robot that is able to help out with daily household chores. Its development focused on giving it the ability to make use of tools, equipment, and appliances that were designed under the assumption of human use. The goal of AR was to be able to silently and autonomously clean within the home. AR can clean up a storage room, sweep and mop floors, remove dishes from the kitchen table and insert them into the dishwasher, open and close doors, and even do the laundry. The robot can even move furniture in order to clean underneath it and when it is finished, put the furniture back in its original location. Its mobility is provided by a two-wheel base that implements a simpler mechanism than the more intricate "leg-based" systems. The robot also has the ability to perform multiple consecutive tasks rather than dealing with each one separately and requiring additional instructions after each completed task.
Technology: The Home Assistant AR stands at 160 cm tall and weighs approximately 130 kg. It uses a total of five cameras and six lasers in order to map out and efficiently navigate the home. A range finder also gives AR the ability to judge distances to obstacles. Based on its self-created 3D geometries of the home, it can execute various complex movements. The robot is equipped with a total of 32 joints (three in the neck and head, seven in each arm, six in each hand, one in the hips, and two in the wheel base) in order to provide it with the flexibility to complete various tasks originally designed for humans. For instance, the neck alone can move in three directions while the arm can move in an impressive seven. It can also assess whether a job it completed was successful, and if determined unsuccessful, repeat the job. The robot can work a total of about 30–60 minutes per charge. Source: www.irt.i.u-tokyo.ac.jp.

System Name: Twendy-One
Developer: Waseda University
Twendy-One (see Figure 4.3) is a type of "human symbiotic" robot that was developed to address the impending labor shortages in the care for aging societies industry. As such, it must incorporate the typical functions carried out by human caregivers including friendly communication, human safety assistance, and dexterous manipulation. The robot was developed with three core principles in mind: Safety, Dependability, and Dexterity. It possesses a unique combination of dexterity with passivity and a high-power output. This allows it to manipulate objects of various shapes with delicacy by passively absorbing external forces generated by their motion. For example, the robot is gentle yet strong enough to support a human getting out of bed but also has the dexterity to remove a piece of toast from the toaster. Other typical tasks carried out by the robot may include fetching things from the fridge, picking things up from the floor, or various cleaning tasks.
Technology: Twendy-One stands at 1.46 m tall and weighs approximately 111 kg. It has a total of 47 degrees of freedom including rotational and directional movements. Its shell is overlaid in a soft silicone skin and equipped with 241 force sensors to detect contact (accidental or intentional) with a human user. This allows the robot to act with care when working with human users as well as adapt to unforeseen collisions instantly and react accordingly. The omnidirectional wheelbase allows the robot to move quicker and more efficient than the traditional bipedal design would. The robot is also equipped with twelve

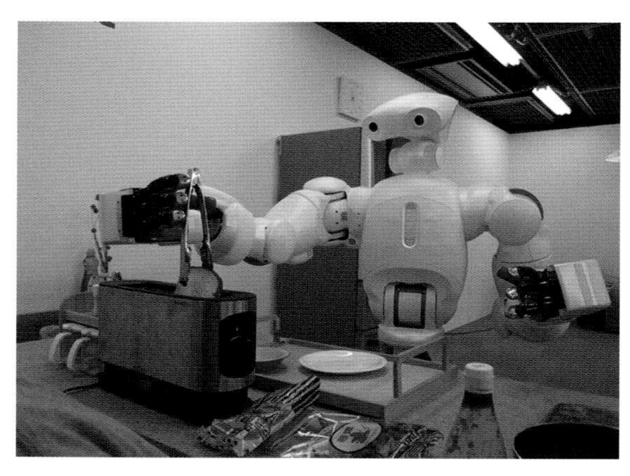

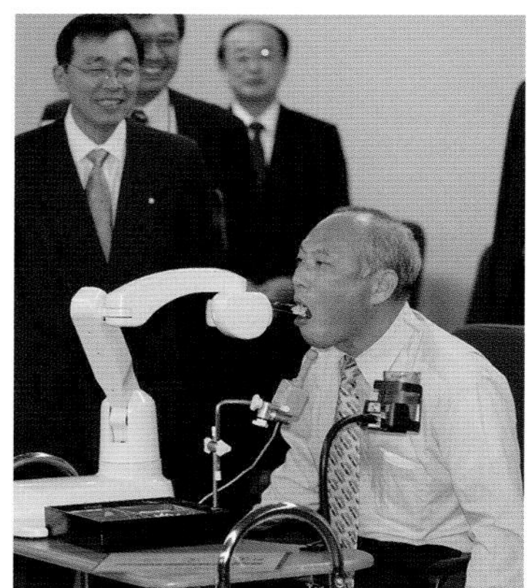

Figure 4.3 Left: Twendy-One.
Source: Shigeki Sugano Lab., Waseda University
Right: My Spoon.
Source: STR/AFP/Getty Images

ultrasonic sensors and a six-axis force sensor to actively detect objects and users and avoid collisions. The robot can operate approximately 15 minutes on a full charge. Source: www.twendyone.com.

System Name: My Spoon
Developer: Secom
My Spoon (see Figure 4.3) is an assistive eating robot. It provides physical assistance for those who would otherwise require human assistance when eating due to some physical disability. It does still require, however, that the user be able to move their head, eat the food off of the spoon, chew, and swallow while sitting in an upright position. My spoon can be used with nearly all types of everyday foods and does not require special food packets for use. The food, should however, be in bite-size pieces as the robot does not include any cutting mechanisms. My Spoon can also be used for liquids such as soft drinks, coffee, tea, or soup. In contrast to most robots, My Spoon is present not only in Japan, but also across Europe.
Technology: My Spoon is 28 cm(W) × 37 cm(D) × 25cm(H) and weighs about 6 kg. It is designed to lie on the table in front of the user. The robot can be operated in one of three modes: manual, semi-automatic, or fully automatic. In manual mode, the user has maximum flexibility and control via a joystick. Using the joystick, the user selects one of four food compartments, fine-tunes the position of the spoon, instructs the spoon to grasp a bite of food, and directs it toward their mouth. In semi-automatic mode, the user simply selects from which compartment they would like a bite and My Spoon automatically picks up a bite from that compartment and brings it to the users' mouth. In the fully automatic mode, with the simple press of a button, My Spoon will automatically select the compartment and will bring a bite of the food up to the users' mouth. Source: www.secom.co.jp/englisch/myspoon

System Name: Maron-1
Developer: Fujitsu
The Maron-1 robot (see Figure 4.4) is a cellular phone–operated system for special patient care, home, and office security. The robot is able to monitor its surroundings, take photos, and

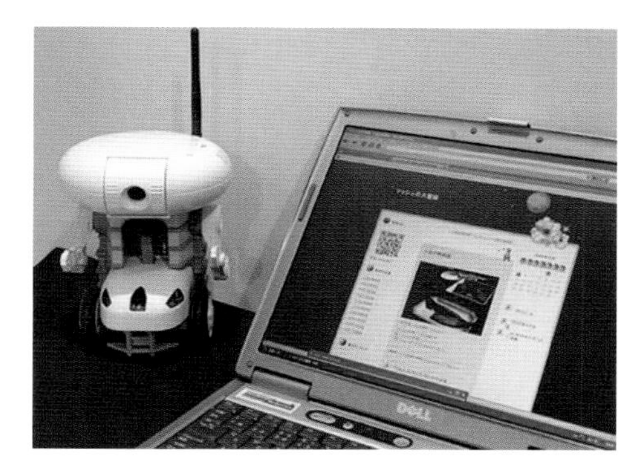

Figure 4.4 The NetTransorWeb.
(Source: Bandai Co., Ltd)

relay the photos to the user via their cell phone. The robot can store the layout of the house or office and if so directed (via a cell phone), can navigate to a specified location while avoiding obstacles and maneuvering across slight changes in floor height. It can also be given a specified "patrol route" to follow and actively monitor. Maron-1 is then able to detect any moving objects that enter its field of view (e.g., an intruder). Maron-1 is also equipped with an infrared remote-control capability that allows it to operate various appliances such as air conditioners, televisions, etc.
Technology: Maron-1 is 32 × 36 × 32 cm and weighs about 5 kg. Its drive mechanism of two powered wheels provides its mobility. It has a head with two cameras that can both pan and tilt to capture as much of the surrounding area as possible. It is also equipped with an infrared sensor/emitter and proximity sensor for appliance operation and obstacle detection. It uses Microsoft's WinCE 3.0 software that allows for its communication with mobile phones. The user interface consists of a touchpad, five menu keys, two function keys, a 10 cm LCD monitor, a speaker, and a microphone. The robot can operate for about 12 hours on a single charge. Source: www.fujitsu.com.

System Name: NetTransorWeb
Developer: Bandai and Evolution Robotics
The NetTransorWeb (Figure 4.4) robot from Bandai and Evolution Robotics was designed as a house robot for families and hobbyists alike. It was also given the quirky ability to blog, which distinguishes it from most other robots. It can even respond to comments left on the blog. For example, it can write context-related replies or take another picture of something in the house, perhaps from a different angle. Aside from this unique feature, the primary purpose of the robot is surveillance. The robot monitors the home and can take pictures of anything that moves (i.e., in the case of an intruder) and immediately alert the owner. It can receive instructions over the internet or autonomously navigate its way around the home.
Technology: The NetTransorWeb is about 190 × 160 × 160 mm big and weighs just 980 grams. Its battery allows for roughly 2.5 hours of operation between charges. It is equipped with cameras, microphones, speakers, and motion sensors. It is also easily connected to the internet or home network over a Wi-Fi connection. The ViPR Vision System from Evolution Robotics provides the robot with a level of intelligence such that it can learn its environment, detect and navigate obstacles, and also perform various tasks including the monitoring and reporting of any unexpected changes in its environment. NetTransorWeb can also collect news

Table 4.2 Overview of the Technology Introduced in this Subsection

System Name	Developer
Panasonic Life Wall	Panasonic
Robot Town & Robot Care	Professor Hasegawa, Kyushu University
Ubiquitous Monitoring System	Hitachi Laboratories
Secure-Life Electronics	Various researchers and companies (e.g., NEC, Toshiba, and Hitachi)
Input Devices & Health Care	Various researchers and companies
Ubiquitous Communication	YRP & UID Center, Ken Sakamura
PARO	AIST, Takanori Shibata
WAKAMURA	Mitsubishi

from the internet (via RSS) and use it to contribute to the blog. Its blogging abilities include uploading, commenting, and answering, often with witty retorts. Unfortunately, the system is not In the market anymore. Source: www.crunchgear.com.

4.2 Social Interaction

In this section, the introduced technology is focused more on the robotics and techniques supporting the care staff in their work. Thereby, the care staff will get released from the physical work and have more time for the social interaction with the elderly. In Table 4.2, a short overview about the robots introduced in this section is presented.

System Name: Panasonic Life Wall
Developer: Panasonic
The "Life Wall TV" from Panasonic transforms an entire wall into an interactive touch screen television that provides large amounts of information and ubiquitous communication. The result is a wall embedded with a digital interface that allows any member of the family to independently access its entertainment, productivity, or communication features. It includes facial and voice recognition software in order to recognize which member of the family is present and will display the graphical user interface (GUI) specific to that person. The display can be made as small or large as the user would like (within the dimensions of the actual screen). The wall can also track your movement throughout the room and, for example, pause your movie while you get up to answer the phone or even have the smaller display follow you around the room. The touch screen allows for stimulating interaction, whether it is for games, system navigation, or any other task. When not in use, the system can be set to a scenic background of the users' choice or it can even disguise itself as a more typical wall by displaying, for example, some bookshelves.
Technology: Panasonic's Life Wall uses a large LCD display. Special facial and voice recognition software allow the system to determine which family member is currently using it and adjust accordingly. The display will show the background, pictures, programs, location of icons and tools, etc., specific to that person. The size, clarity, and interaction ability of the system take photo viewing, videoconferences, and computer games into another dimension. The Life Wall is also equipped with "Wireless HD" abilities to incorporate the internet into any of these aforementioned features. Source: www.panasonic.com/cesshow/.

System Name: Robot Town & Robot Care
Developer: Professor Hasegawa, Kyushu University
Robot Town (see Figure 4.5) is based on the premise of robots' limitations in recognizing the environment they are in, reacting to it, and learning from these experiences. This project looks to demonstrate how robots can be more efficient in the future. According to Professor Hasegawa, in order for this to happen, the environments must be structured in a way that they become more recognizable to the robots. In this way, the necessary complexities are removed from the robot itself and transferred into the intelligent systems comprising the surrounding environment. These intelligent systems supply to the robot information such as location – the location of other robots – and direction for action. This approach was further developed into a "Town Management System" (TMS) in which the city is in constant interaction with the robots. The robots are provided with specific relevant information and duties. Thanks to the TMS, it is no longer required that the robot itself be equipped with these high-performance systems but can rather rely on the infrastructure already in place. This allows the robots to be more mobile. At the same time, 1,000 RFID tags dispersed throughout the town provide the robots with real time information on their precise location and state of their surroundings.
Technology: The TMS was designed specifically with senior homes in mind. The system was also tested in this setting. It was used to support the nursing staff in the home. The test setting covered 1700 m^2 and was equipped with a video monitoring system. Source: www.kyushu-u-ac.jp/english/.

System Name: Ubiquitous Monitoring System
Developer: Hitachi Laboratories
The concept of "Monitoring Systems" displays not only the instantaneous health parameters (i.e., vital signs), but also provides a continuous monitoring of these parameters as well as

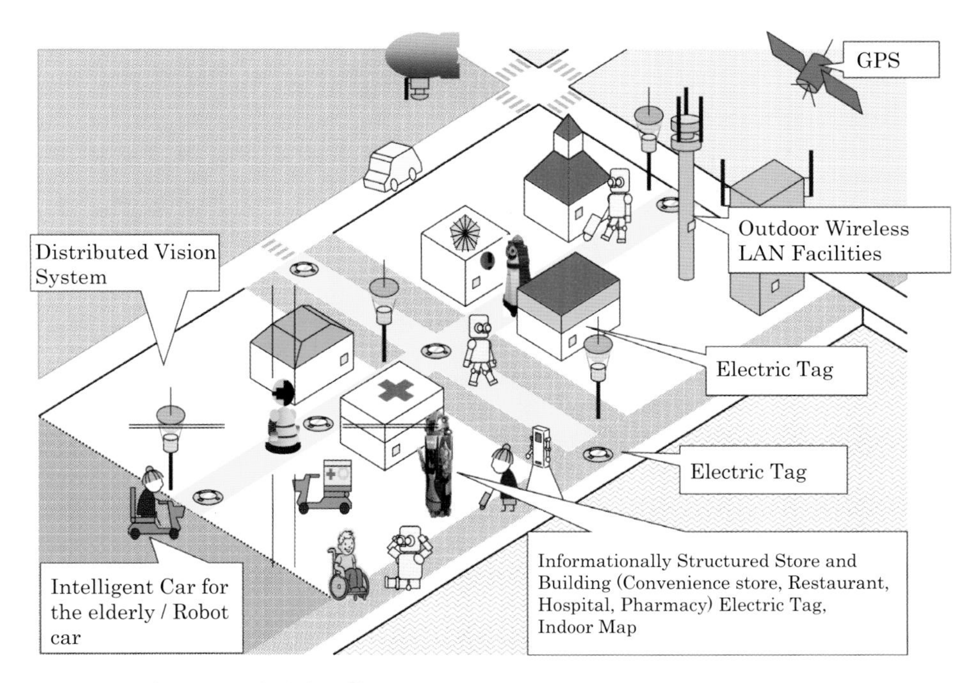

Figure 4.5 Robot Town & Robot Care.
Source: Ken'ichi Morooka, Kyushu University

considers the future trends and implications of any perceived patterns. If a problem is detected with one of the monitored users, the system can take the necessary actions including alerting a caregiver or emergency services. The system is able to actively track and monitor a variety of users and their various performances in their daily routines in real time. For example, parents could monitor their children as the children make their way to school to ensure that they arrive there safely. The system uses "Peer-to-Peer" (P2P) technology. This type of system can also be used for the tracking of everyday objects such as wallets or backpacks, and should these items be misplaced, can notify the user on their location. During the development of the system, an emphasis was placed on their universal use in the context of demographic change. This system could be used in a variety of different settings including public (e.g., by the police) and private (e.g., in the home setting).

System Name: Secure-Life Electronics
Developer: Various researchers and companies (e.g., NEC, Toshiba, and Hitachi)
The goal of the Center of Excellence (COE) programs is to further develop MST-based technologies. This is important as it allows the improvement of the quality of life of those individuals that may require assistance in carrying out their necessary daily activities. When developing these technologies, it is important to adopt a universal approach in order not to exclude populations from different cultures, backgrounds, economic standing, etc. These specialized technologies are used for social interaction as well as technical and physical infrastructure and therefore positively influence the everyday lives of the aging population and their caregivers. As these technologies often include multi-faceted aspects, developers with specializations covering a wide variety of backgrounds are required. This is true for many technologies presented in this book and facilitates the important synergetic technology transfer between fields.
Technologies included within these systems include:

- Sensory systems
- Information processing networks
- Actuators
- Devices with various application cases
- Systems integration
- Bio-sensory systems
- "Right-Brain Computing"

Source: www.u-tokyo.ac.jp/coe/.

System Name: Input Devices & Health Care
Developer: Various researchers and companies
According to the national "u-Japan" strategy, "ubiquitous" communication and specifically the user interfaces required for these communication devices, will play an increasing role in the future. This is as a result of the significant demographic changes being experienced by many developed countries, specifically in Asia (i.e., Japan) and Europe (i.e., Germany). The interdisciplinary field of microsystems technology is used in various areas of the development of these technologies. Research and experimentation on topics such as sensory systems, actuating systems, bio-MEMS, insect-based robots, etc., is ongoing and will provide significant advancements in this field in the not too distant future. However, a clear focus will remain on different interfaces allowing seamless and intuitive human-machine interaction.
Technologies in this field include:

- Wearable Input Devices
- Mobile Pointing Shoes
- Systems that provide health data
- Organic Semiconductor-based strain sensors

Source: www.leopard.t.u-tokyo.ac.jp/research.html.

System Name: Ubiquitous Communication
Developer: YRP & UID Center, Ken Sakamura
In Tokyo's business, entertainment district and the most famous shopping quarter in Japan, Ginza, a large-scale experiment involving the use of RFID tags is ongoing. Approximately 10,000 RFID tags are distributed throughout the district and are interconnected with various Bluetooth systems, internet servers, special reading devices, and information systems. The experiment is being made multi-lingual allowing non-native people and businesses to also take part. This large-scale Tokyo Ubiquitous Network project uses an extensive RFID network structure in order to provide users the ability to accurately determine their exact location and easily plan their navigation through the large urban center. Tokyo's governor, Shintaro Ishihara, inaugurated the experiment at the opening event in Ginza. As each building contains several stores, bars, and clubs, finding the right one can often be difficult. With this new technique, a push of a button will allow you to immediately find your exact location and in which direction you must go to reach your desired destination.
Technology: From the beginning of December 2008, RFID tags were dispersed throughout the entire quarter on buildings, street corners, street lamps, and in bars and shops. Reading devices with a 3.5 inch OLED display allowed users to read the RFID tags and obtain location data and directions. Each RFID tag has a specific code indicating its specific location. This data is wirelessly transmitted over WLAN to a centralized server. The server transmits the desired data (i.e., location, specific directions) back to the user's reading device. This experiment, managed by the Tokyo Ubiquitous Computing Center, was a joint venture between the Japanese government, the city of Tokyo, the Ministry of Agriculture Infrastructure and Transport (MILT) as well as several other additional companies. Similar experiments are currently ongoing in other Japanese cities.

System Name: Interaction: PARO
Developer: AIST, Takanori Shibata
The positive influence animals have on the elderly or those suffering psychological disabilities is already well known. However, the integration of living animals into these homecare situations is often difficult and impractical. To address this, AIST has developed PARO (see Figure 4.6), an advanced interactive robot able to provide the documented benefits of animal companionship. The robot addresses concerns such as misbehavior, hygiene, noises, and smells that may accompany living animals. PARO has been found to reduce stress in both patients and caregivers and even stimulates interaction between the two. By interacting with the users (speaking with them, listening to them, and responding to their touch), PARO effectively simulates an animal companion and provides direct benefits such as; increased activity in social interaction, including visual, verbal, and physical. Additionally, PARO also ensures increased levels of both motivation and relaxation.
Technology: PARO is equipped with five different types of sensors: tactile, light, audition, temperature, and posture. This allows the robot to actively perceive people and its environment. The tactile sensor allows it to detect touch movements such as stroking or petting while the posture sensor allows it to detect when and in what position it is being held. The audio sensor allows it to detect voices (and the direction of their origin), greetings, and compliments. PARO is also able to learn and remember actions; for example, if it is stroked each time after a certain movement, it will try to repeat that movement in order to be stroked again. These sensors and movements allow the robot to respond to users as if it was alive, even mimicking the voice of a genuine baby seal. Source: www.AIST.jp.

System Name: Interaction and Information: WAKAMARU
Developer: Mitsubishi
The WAKAMARU (see Figure 4.6) robot from Mitsubishi was primarily developed as a companion and helper to the elderly and disabled. It is not, however, used for housework

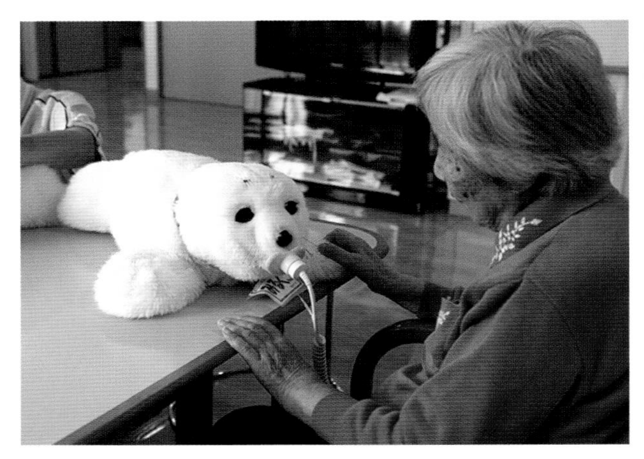

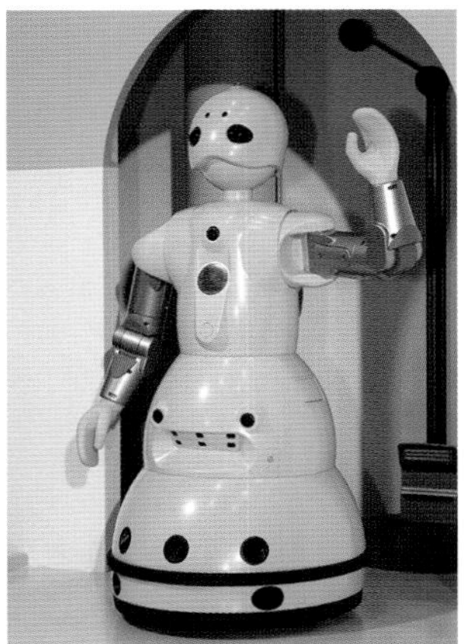

Figure 4.6 Left: PARO.
Source: Yamaguchi Haruyoshi/Corbis via Getty Images
Right: WAKAMARU.
Source: YOSHIKAZU TSUNO/AFP/Getty Images

chores such as vacuum cleaning and unloading of the dishwasher. Instead, the robot acts as a sort of secretary for the user. It can move, follow the user around, take notes, and remind them of appointments. It can also provide the user with updated information from the internet, such as the weather forecast, and give advice accordingly such as what types of clothes to wear and to remember their umbrella. It can also be used to ensure that users remember such vital tasks as taking their daily medication.
Technology: The robot stands approximately 1 m in height and weighs 30 kg. It has a flat circular base on which it can roll around with a speed of up to 1 km/h. Facial recognition software allows the robot to recognize and remember up to 10 faces. It is equipped with touch and motion sensors, two video cameras, and four microphones to autonomously interact with its environment. Its ultrasound capabilities also allow it to recognize, detect, and avoid obstacles. Using this knowledge, it creates a plan of all the rooms in the house and is constantly aware of its own location. This allows the robot to know where to go and how to get there. The software is Linux-based and includes a vocabulary of over 10,000 words. This makes the robot fully adequate to converse with human users. The robot is constantly connected to the internet and can readily answer any knowledge-based question. It can recall up to 10 people and remember their daily routines or preferences. It also saves all dates, appointments, etc. it is told and can provide reminders as the time approaches. It can operate for approximately 2 hours before requiring charging, which it can also initiate by itself. Source: www.mhi.co.jp/kobe/wakamaru.

4.3 Health and Wellness

In this section, technology and robots that support the hygienic and recovery processes of elderly and disabled people are introduced to the reader. Table 4.3 gives an overview of the technologies described here.

Table 4.3 Overview of the Technologies Introduced in this Chapter

System Name	Developer
Intelligent Toilet	Toto and Daiwa House Industry
Bathing Machine HIRB	Sanyo
Bathing Machine Santelubain 999	AVANT
Health Phone	Fujitsu and NTT DoCoMo
Hitachi Genki Chip	Hitachi
Ubiquitous Communication	YRP & UID Center, Ken Sakamura
Rehabilitation Suit REALIVE™	Panasonic, Activelink, Kobe Gakuin University
RIBA	Institute of Physical and Chemical Research (RIKEN), Tokai Rubber Industries (TRI)
Robotic Bed	Panasonic

System Name: Intelligent Toilet
Developer: Toto and Daiwa House Industry
This fully automatic toilet eliminates the need for users to manually perform tasks such as opening and closing the cover, as well as flushing the toilet in hopes of improving cleanliness. The toilet is also equipped with various health-monitoring functions, such as measuring the sugar levels in urine, blood pressure, body fat, and weight. The built-in urine analyzer is implemented into the toilet in a non-invasive manner, and the device automatically cleans itself after each use. The second version of the toilet is also able to measure the temperature of urine as well as monitor the menstruation cycle of women. The goal of this project is to provide users with the ability to have automated check-ups done in the comfort of their own home and reduce unnecessary trips to the doctor.
Technology: The intelligent toilet (visible in Figure 4.7) collects 5 cm^3 of urine from the user for analysis purposes. This sample collector is able to automatically clean itself after each use. The blood pressure monitor is within arm's reach of the toilet and the scales in front of the sink weigh the user as they wash their hands. The results of the bathroom medical are then transferred to a home network and analyzed in a computer spreadsheet. This allows the users to adjust their lifestyle based on their personal analyzed data. For example, they can alter their diet to reduce their sugar intake or increase daily activity in order to achieve a healthier body mass index. The system can also advise the user if a trip to the actual doctor's office should be made. Source: www.daiwahouse.co.jp, www.engadget.com.

System Name: Bathing Machine HIRB
Developer: Sanyo
The "Human In Roll-lo Bathing" (HIRB, visible in Figure 4.7) unit from Sanyo is a compact automatic bathing machine geared toward elderly users. The unit is an improvement over Sanyo's first attempt at such a product, the "Ultrasonic Bath" which was a concept displayed at the 1970 World Expo in Osaka, Japan. The original concept was nearly 2 meters tall and required a ladder to reach the elevated bathing capsule. The HIRB unit is more practically designed and is geared toward an institutional setting such as care homes for the elderly. The user sits in a chair that rolls backward into the bathtub. The clam-like shell of the bathtub then closes around the user, leaving only their head and shoulders exposed. The wash cycle, consisting of soap and rinse cycles, operates fully automatically. The machine is able to complete everything except the shampooing and washing of hair, which must still be done manually. The HIRB unit assists the nursing staff by automatically carrying out work that can

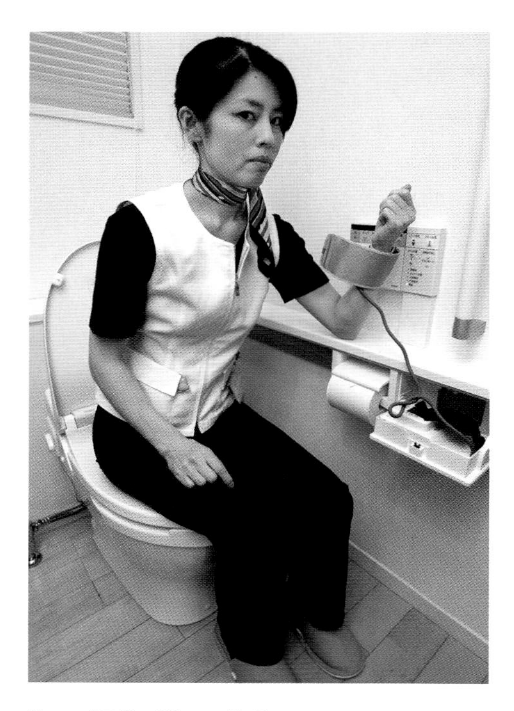

Figure 4.7 Intelligent Toilet.
Source: Getty Images

be both time consuming and strenuous on the body while preserving the privacy of the patient. Source: Sanyo Japan.

System Name: Bathing Machine Santelubain 999
Developer: AVANT
The Santelubain 999 allows the user to climb in and rest in a lying position while undergoing an automated bathing experience. In addition to the necessary bathing functions, the system also possesses some beauty and therapeutic abilities. Some of the options in the system include:

- Shampoo and washing
- Infrared heating and steam treatment
- Audio therapy
- Aromatherapy
- Seaweed wrap
- Body lotion

Following the bathing or treatment session, the Santelubain 999 is also able to automatically clean and sterilize itself. Source: www.avant.ne.jp.

System Name: Health Phone
Developer: Fujitsu and NTT DoCoMo
At the Japanese "Wireless Expo 2008," Fujitsu and NTT DoCoMo presented their "Health Phone" geared toward aging societies. With the F884iES, users are able to check their heart rate wherever they are.

The F884iES can also connect with various Bluetooth or Infrared enabled Tanita products (Tanita holds approximately 50 percent of the Japanese market share for fitness and health scales) such as body fat measurement, blood pressure measurement, and pacemakers. Using these devices, various health data can be saved to a "health calendar" or even sent to the user's doctor, fitness club, dietician, etc.
Technology: The F884iES is equipped with, among other features, a 2 Megapixel camera, dual color display, a media player, high speed internet connection, and expandable hard drive storage. Special features of the phone include a built-in pacemaker and an integrated pulse measurer as well as a second camera.
Users measure their pulse using a method called pulse oximetry in which a small infrared light is used to measure the pulse through the tip of the finger. In addition to Fujitsu's F884iES, Sharp has a similar phone (SH706IW) with many similar features. Source: www.funponsel.com.

System Name: Hitachi Genki Chip
Developer: Hitachi
Much time and many resources are used in the complicated and lengthy process of blood analysis. This problem is made worse by aging populations as senior citizens often require these analyses more often. This can result in the needs of other patients, who may be in more immediate danger, often becoming delayed or overlooked.
The Genki Chip from Hitachi makes it possible to summarize important health data, test results, and medical history of a patient in one compact chip. This gives doctors and physicians immediate access to all of the information they need before they can administer any treatment to a patient. It also allows for a reduction in costly or elaborate laboratory analysis as the care giving staff also have access to necessary patient information.
Technology: Mental stress can impose a negative effect on the immune system just as with the endocrine system. For this reason, it is possible to assess the psychological state of a patient using a chemical analysis of the blood. The Genki chip enables this analysis to take place quickly and efficiently as it records and stores the analysis results. Using this rapid analysis technique allows faster intervention by physicians and can allow patients to be treated faster and safer in the event of a sudden change of condition. Source: Hitachi Hybrid Network Co. Ltd.

System Name: Rehabilitation Suit REALIVE™
Developer: Panasonic, Activelink, Kobe Gakuin University
The REALIVE suit was developed as an assistive rehabilitation system for people that have suffered a stroke and have lost the ability to move upper limbs on one side of their body due to paralysis. The suit works by detecting movement in the unaffected side of the body and assisting the user to mirror that movement on the paralyzed side of the body. This concept is a direct result of medical research that found that "visual feedback of the movement and intensive use of the affected upper limbs can stimulate the cerebral nerves – that go off-line due to cerebrovascular accidents – and improve rehabilitation". The design focused on developing a suit that was "visible but invisible", looked and felt good to wear while at the same time maintaining the highest level of user safety. The robotic suit was developed for rehabilitation in the hospital or institutional setting. However, Panasonic hopes to make the suit affordable enough for home use with time.
Technology: The robotic REALIVE suit senses movement in the unaffected side of the body through a series of sensors. The sensors then send the signals to the artificial pneumatic "rubber muscles" wrapped around the affected limbs or muscles on the other side of the body. These "muscles" assist the user in mimicking that movement on the affected side of the body

and this movement helps to facilitate their rehabilitation. The sensors and artificial muscles are controlled via compressed air. They are linked to a compressed air unit that also displays the number of times the muscles have been moved. The suit underwent clinical testing at Hyogo Hospital in 2009. Source: www.panasonic.co.jp/corp/news.

System Name: RIBA
Developer: Institute of Physical and Chemical Research (RIKEN), Tokai Rubber Industries (TRI)
The Robot for Interactive Body Assistance (RIBA, visible in Figure 4.8) is an assistive robot that can help nursing staff lift and transport patients. The robot can assist with the difficult transition transport required to and from the patient's bed or wheelchair, or also to and from the toilet. At the time of its development, it was claimed to be the first robot that could safely and efficiently lift up or sit down a human being. The robot is limited to a weight capacity of 61 kg (134 lbs). RIBA is the second-generation robot following its predecessor, RI-MAN, which was hampered with concerns over limited safety and performance functionality. Considering the number of times each patient must be lifted and moved each day, RIBA proves to be a valuable asset. The robot not only reduces the strain on caregivers' backs by completing the lifting actions for them, but also increases the safety of the patients that must be transported.
Technology: RIBA weighs about 180 kg, stands about 1.4 m tall, and moves around on an omnidirectional circular base equipped with omni-wheels. Its ability to safely and efficiently lift and transport humans comes from its strong human-like arms and pinpoint accuracy. The robot is guided by high-accuracy tactile sensors in order to determine in what position the human is in and how best to lift them. It is equipped with special joints and link lengths optimized for lifting humans. This system was developed by pairing RIKEN's control, sensor, and image processing with TRI's strength in material and structural design. The robot is able to detect and respond to basic verbal commands from nurses with its two microphones and two cameras. The robot is powered by a DC motor and can operate for one hour per charge. Source: http://rtc.nagoya.riken.jp/RIBA.

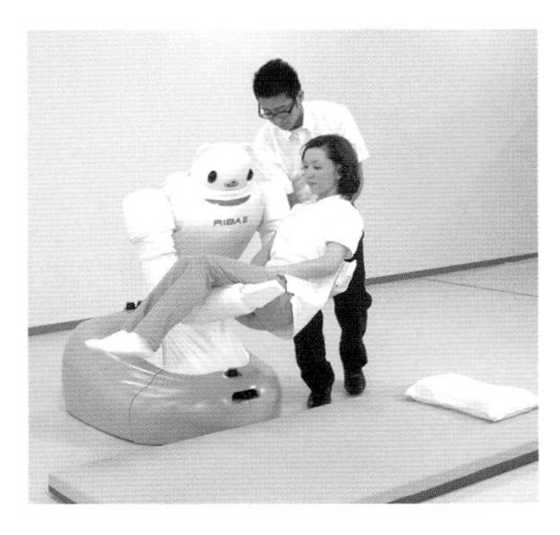

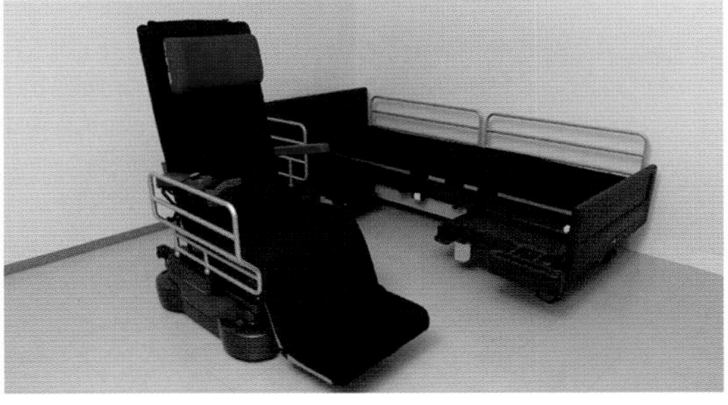

Figure 4.8 Left: RIBA.
Source: RIKEN RTC
Right: Robotic Bed.
Source: Panasonic

System Name: Robotic Bed
Developer: Panasonic
The Robotic Bed (depicted in Figure 4.8) from Panasonic was developed to assist with the transition of elderly patients from the wheelchair and into the bed. Similar to other technologies presented in this book, Panasonic's first attempt at this used strong robotic arms to assist in the lifting of patients. The Robotic bed, however, is a wheelchair-bed combination that negates the need for patient transportation as the wheelchair can transform into a bed and vice versa. This also minimizes strain on care staff as the assistance required for this transformation is minimal. The mattress splits in half – with one half remaining as part of the bed, and the other half forming the shape of the wheelchair. A patient simply needs to shift to one side of the bed, and after a few remote-controlled adjustments, can sit upright in a modified wheelchair.
Technology: The Robotic Bed can be controlled automatically with a simple remote control. It then completes the transformation to bed or wheelchair automatically. The power-assisted tilting of the bed helps to optimally distribute the weight of the user in order to prevent them from the discomfort of slipping during transformation as well as relieving stress that may build up due to extended periods of sitting. Source: https://news.panasonic.com/global/press/data/en090918-2/en090918-2.html.

4.4 Information and Learning

In this section, two Information and Learning platforms as shown in Table 4.4 are introduced.

System Name: EZ Touch Remote Control
Developer: Panasonic
The EZ Touch Remote Control (see Figure 4.9) is a product that in coordination with the "u-Japan" Strategy, is aimed at promoting access to various networks, technologies, and therefore services to the general and specifically, aging populations. With this device, Panasonic is looking to modernize the remote control with their new innovative design. Instead of looking down at the remote control in order to locate the correct buttons, this design displays the touch screen on the televisions screen, where the user wants to look anyway. The remote detects whether a user is right-handed or left-handed and adjusts the layout accordingly, placing important buttons within thumb's reach. The onscreen display can be set to be large and simplistic, specifically tailored to those hesitant to embrace novel technologies or those with a problematic eyesight.
Technology: The EZ Touch Remote Control is equipped with two touchpads. The dual touchpads allow for multi-touch user manipulation which allows for a variety of gestures that can control aspects such as zooming and scrolling. The remote control still has physical buttons at the center for quick control of volume, channels, and power. Source: http://Panasonic.co.jp.corp.

Table 4.4 Overview of the Technology Introduced in this Chapter

System Name	Developer
EZ Touch Remote Control	Panasonic
Dr. Kawashima's Brain Training	Nintendo, Dr. Ryuta Kawashima

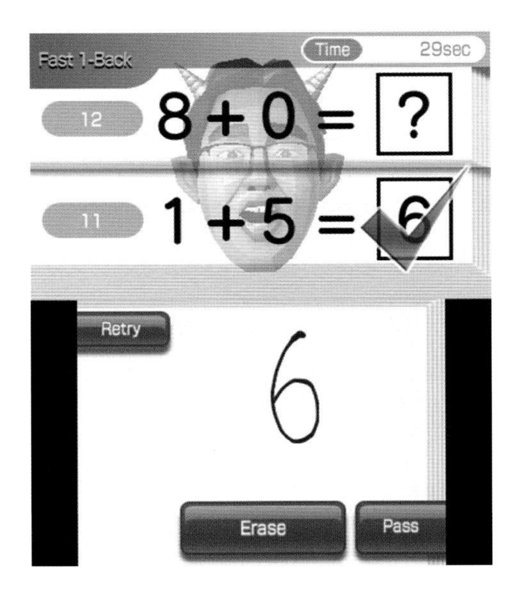

Figure 4.9 Dr. Kawashima's Brain Training.
Source: Nintendo

System Name: Dr. Kawashima's Brain Training
Developer: Nintendo, Dr. Ryuta Kawashima
Dr. Kawashima's Brain Training (shown in Figure 4.9), also known as Brain Age: "Train Your Brain in Minutes a Day!", is a video game for the Nintendo DS that uses puzzles and various types of problems to stimulate the brain. Although the game has not been scientifically tested and validated, it is 'inspired' by Dr. Kawashima's research in the field of neuroscience. It allows users that may suffer from decreased brain activity from age, diet, sickness, poor sleep, etc., to evaluate the state of their brain and 'train' it back to health through daily exercising. After completing any puzzle, the user is informed of the 'age' of their brain based on how fast they were able to complete it. They are also given tips for improvement. In total, there are five modes of play: Brain Age Check, Training, Quick Play, Download, and Sudoku. Each mode of play includes a variety of different games, puzzles, and tasks for the user to choose from.
Technology: The game is designed for daily usage with only a few minutes each day required to improve your brain and lower your 'Brain Age'. Daily tasks include mental arithmetic, counting, speed reading, or syllable counting. The Nintendo DS system is used as a sort of digital book where one side is used for display and the other side for user input, depending on whether the use is left or right-handed. It has a touchscreen and microphone to capture user input. Although Nintendo stresses that they are in the entertainment business only and make no claims about the games effectiveness on improving brain activity, the game is recommended by many neurologists to patients suffering from dementia or Alzheimer's. Source: www.braintraining.com.au/.

4.5 Working

In this section, information and communication system which support either the physical, or mental work e.g., by finding the correct path or reducing the force on the

Table 4.5 Overview of the Technologies Introduced in this Subsection

System Name	Developer
Roppongi Hills R-clicks	NTT DoCoMo Inc.
Stride Management Assist and Bodyweight Support Assist	Honda
Brain-Machine Interface: Honda, Toyota	Honda, Toyota, ART, and Shimadzu Corp.

muscles by wearable robots are presented. In Table 4.5, an overview about the technology introduced in this section is given.

System Name: Roppongi Hills R-clicks
Developer: NTT DoCoMo Inc.
NTT DoCoMo Inc. began the development of their Roppongi Hills R-clicks system in 2003 (see Figure 4.10). R-clicks was developed as an information service to provide users with detailed information regarding their environment via their cell phones. The system works using RFID tags. It was first tested with the Mori Building Co. Ltd. complex in Roppongi Hills, Tokyo. The first participants were each given an RFID tag reader and from this, the system could determine their exact location. More than 4500 RFID tags were dispersed throughout the area. The system could then send the desired information to the user's cell phone as they move through the various complexes, stores, hotels, and entertainment venues of the area. The information was accessed on their cell phone via iMode capabilities. In some cases, the cell phone itself could even be modified into a scanner and eliminate the need for a secondary scanning device.
Technology: There are three detailed scenarios on how a user might benefit from R-clicks:

1. Koko Dake (Environment Information)
   While standing in any of the 20 or more zones of Roppongi Hills, users can scan an RFID tag and immediately receive detailed information generated specifically for them regarding their environment.
2. Mite Toru (Visit and Listen)
   While standing in front of a display board, the user can receive information regarding specific products, services, etc., related to their current environment
3. Buratto (Tour)
   While moving around, the user can receive current information regarding their environment, including when they are entering into a new zone and what attractions may be within this zone.

Source: www.nttdocomo.com

System Name: Stride Management Assist and Bodyweight Support Assist
Developer: Honda
Honda began their research into electronic assistive walking devices in 1999 by initiating research, various studies of human walking, and the development of many different conceptual variations. Much of the research was devoted to the development of Honda's signature humanoid robot, ASIMO, but inadvertently led to many different spinoff stand-alone technologies with real-world practical use cases. Two of these by-products are the 'Stride Management Assist' and the 'Bodyweight Support Assist'. Both systems are 'worn' by the user providing joint and muscle support where required. The Stride Management Assist uses a motor to assist the user to lift each leg at the thigh while walking. It is designed for people who may have weakened leg muscles but are still able to walk and lengthens their stride while regulating their walking pace. The Bodyweight

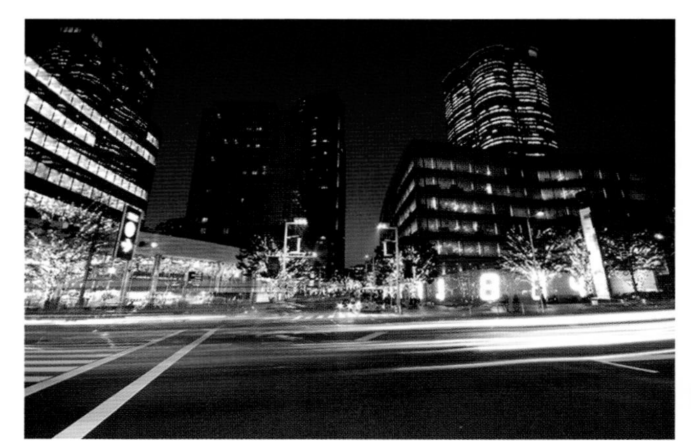

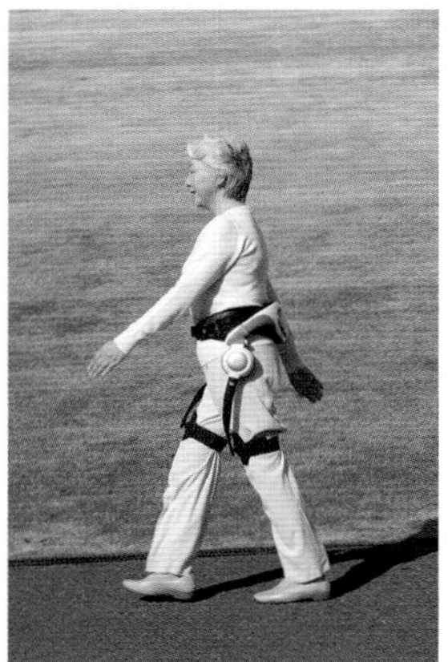

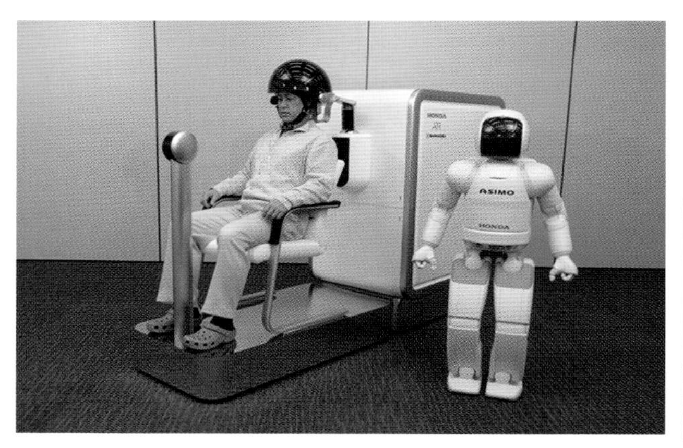

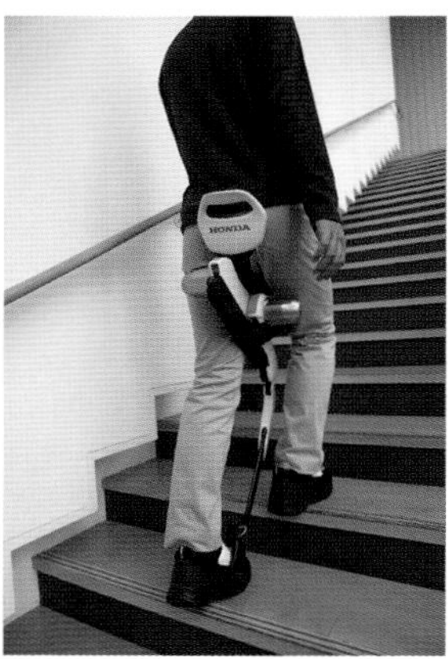

Figure 4.10 Top left: Roppongi Hills.
Bottom left: Brain-Machine Interface.
Top right: Stride Management Assist.
Bottom right: Bodyweight Support Assist.
Source: Honda

Support Assist allows users to walk while carrying a 'lighter' body. The system supports the user's upper body in order to reduce stress on the legs while walking, going up or down the stairs, and in semi-crouching positions.

Technology: Both systems (see Figure 4.10) use a series of sensors to detect the motions of the user's walking. An integrated computer uses this data to control the light metal braces and move seamlessly with the user. The 'Stride Management Assist' uses a compact DC motor and the system is relatively light at only 2.8 kg, including the lithium-ion batteries. The batteries have a run-time of approximately 2 hours at a walking pace of 4.5 km/h. The 'Bodyweight Support Assist' uses sensors in the shoes to determine the desired movements of both the left and right legs. The system supports the user and reduces the load on their legs while walking, climbing, or even just standing. The system weighs 6.5 kg and also uses lithium-ion batteries that give it a run-time of approximately 2 hours. Source: http://world.honda.com/news.

System Name: Brain-Machine Interface
Developer: Honda, Toyota, ART, and Shimadzu Corp.
The "Brain-Machine Interface" (BMI, visible Figure 4.10) is the first example in the futuristic field of 'thought-controlled' robots. The system was developed at the BSI-Toyota Collaboration Center (BTCC), which was established by the Japanese government and their industrial partners. The system processes the users' brain activity, which can then direct the robot to move left, right, or straight ahead. There is no need for any implants or invasive surgery as the system utilizes a series of sensors placed on the users' skull. An emergency stop feature has been implemented by means of the user 'puffing out their cheek'. Practically, this can be applied to control wheelchair movements regardless of someone's physical inabilities.
Technology: The technology of using brain activity to control a machine is not entirely new, however, Honda and Toyota have found a way to reduce the reaction time of the system down to a mere thousandth of a second, a vast improvement over preceding systems. It accomplishes this by measuring the electrical activity in the user's brain via electroencephalography (EEG) data gathered from a series of five sensors placed over the motor-movement areas of the brain. These electrical impulses from the user's brain are picked up and analyzed by an on-board laptop, which then translates them to movement. The system also learns the 'thinking' patterns of the user and can adjust in order to improve accuracy to levels of 9 percent. Source: www.akihabaranews.com.

4.6 Mobility

Mobility means life quality, especially for the diseased and fragile people, e.g., the elderly. Today's technology allows us to travel fast over kilometers by train, car, or airplane. However, the large distances are not critical, the short distances are the main problem. Supporting devices like rolators can help, but have their limits (e.g., at stairs). Therefore, researchers investigated the use of wearable robots and new mobility concepts, in order to keep the fragile and elderly mobile and thereby independent. In this subsection, the mobility aids of the Table 4.6 are introduced to the reader.

System Name: HAL-5 Enhanced Mobility Suit
Developer: Cyberdyne, Tsukauba University, Prof. Sankai's Team, Daiwa House
The Hybrid Assistive Limb (HAL-5) (see Figure 4.11) is a robotic suit that is worn in order to enhance the user's strength and mobility. The suit was designed to assist elderly users with daily activities, but additional applications of the suit include assistive rehabilitation, assistance to paralyzed individuals by enabling mobility, assistance to nurses and factory workers in strenuous activities, and even assistance with rescue and clean-up efforts following a natural disaster. Interested in robots from a young age, Professor Sankai began developing HAL immediately after receiving his Ph.D. in robotics in 1990. HAL-5 is the fifth iteration of the system and is unique in its completeness and already enjoys widespread use.
Technology: When a person wishes to move a certain part of their body, nerve signals are sent from the brain to that part of the body. When this happens, small bio signals can actually be detected on the skin at that part of the body the person wishes to move. The suit uses electrodes mounted on the user's skin in order to analyse and detect these muscle movements. The system then uses these signals to compliment the user's motion, enhancing the user's strength by up to five times what it normally would be. The suit is powered by a 100-volt battery pack that is mounted at the user's waist. It includes both a user-activated "voluntary control system" and a "robotic autonomous control system" for motion support. Source: www.cyberdyne.jp.

Table 4.6 Overview about the Mobility Aids Introduced in this Subsection

System Name	Developer
HAL-5 Enhanced Mobility Suit	Cyberdyne, Tsukauba University, Prof. Sankai's Team, Daiwa House
WL-16R3 Robot Legs / Walking Wheelchair	Waseda University, Prof. Takanishi's Team
i-foot / Toyota Mobility Suit	Toyota
i-Real	Toyota
i-Swing	Toyota
Wheelchair Robot	Toyota
RCAST Group: Space Technology for Rehabilitation Science	JAXA Institute
i-Road (Personal Mobility)	Toyota
Toyota Mobility Assistance Program	Toyota
Toyota RIN Interior	Toyota
Toyota Sustainable Mobility WINGLET	Toyota
AIST Intelligent Wheelchair	AIST, Yutaka Satoh
Suzuki SSC	Suzuki
Universal Vehicle RODEM	VEDA International R&D Center, TMSUK Co.
City-Car PIVO	Nissan, Takashi Murakimi, Cyberdyne, Tsukuba University

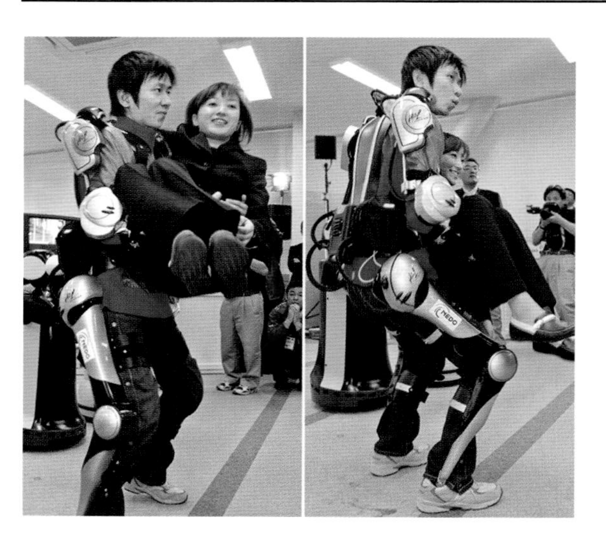

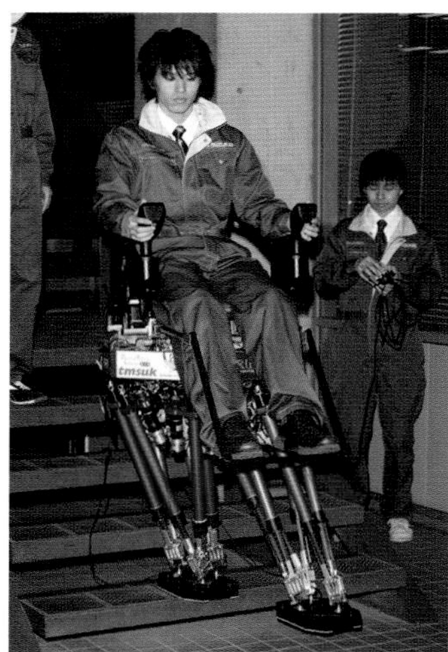

Figure 4.11 Left: HAL-5 Enhanced Mobility Suit.
Source: YOSHIKAZU TSUNO/AFP/Getty Images
Right: WL-16R3 Robot Legs.
Source: Atsuo Takanishi, Waseda University

System Name: WL-16R3 Robot Legs / Walking Wheelchair
Developer: Waseda University, Prof. Takanishi's Team
The WL-16R3 (see Figure 4.11), also known as the 'Walking Wheelchair', was designed as a mobility solution for those that are unable to walk. The design team wanted to address the

shortcomings of alternative solutions (e.g., use of Segway still requiring user to stand, or limiting terrain such as stairs for wheelchairs). The result was a bipedal robot that the user sits atop and controls using a pair of joysticks, one for each hand. This allows the physically disabled users a more flexible range of mobility from a sitting position. The user is even able to safely navigate stairs while sitting atop the WL-16R3.
Technology: The WL-16R3 stands at approximately 122 cm (4 feet) tall and weighs about 68 kg (150 lbs). It is controlled by a single user via two joysticks. In addition to navigating uneven terrain, the robot is also capable of vertical movements, for example, in the ascent or descent of stairs. The legs of the robot take the form of telescoping poles, which allow for the required vertical movements. The poles are fixed to flat plates that act as the 'feet' of the system. The robot is battery controlled and uses pneumatic cylinders for control of the legs. It uses a total of 12 actuators to move forwards, backward, or sideways and can accommodate a user weight of up to 60 kg (130 lbs). The robot can even adjust to the users shifting in the chair to ensure a smooth and comfortable ride. The typical walking stride of the robot is approximately 30 cm but the robot can stretch its legs up to 136 cm apart. Source: www.waseda.jp.

System Name: i-foot / Toyota Mobility Suit
Developer: Toyota
Toyota, widely known for their automotive business, is constantly planning for future business streams in hopes of leading the next product revolution. One of these views involves humans residing, working, and living within immense housing complexes and roofed metropolises. In this scenario, due to spatial and environmental constraints, the traditional automobile may no longer exist in its current form. For this reason, Toyota has developed a series of "i-units" to address the need for futuristic transportation. The basic concept behind the "i-foot" (see Figure 4.12), or Toyota Mobility Suit, is the extension of human ability. These units act as personal transportation vehicles and work together with other household robots in order to optimize usability. In this context, the system can be seen as especially beneficial for the elderly and/or physically disabled. The connection is clear, for someone who spends their entire life being carried around in a personal vehicle, even a trip to the refrigerator proves exhausting.
Technology: The inspiration behind Toyota's "i-foot" comes from their interpretation of bird legs. These legs are mounted on the chassis, and together, provide the movement for the system. The egg-shaped body consists of a bowl-shaped seat that lights up and has steering modules for the operation of the robots. Steering is made possible through the use of an instrument panel and joystick on the right side of the unit. The entire unit stands at approximately 2.36 m tall and weighs about 200 kg. It can accommodate passengers up to a weight of 60 kg and has a maximum speed of roughly 1.35 km/h. Source: www.toyota.co.jp/en.

System Name: i-Real
Developer: Toyota
With the "i-Real", Toyota presents another approach in the direction of ecological and sustainable mobility for future transportation requirements. Despite the futuristic design, Toyota is convinced that single-user vehicles are an integral part of an emission free future for transportation. The concept of the "i-Real" (see Figure 4.12) is based on previously developed mobility studies of single passenger vehicles completed by Toyota (namely the "i-unit" and the "i-Swing"). So far, the "i-Real" is not ready for mass production, but Toyota's support for individual transportation for the transportation of the future is clear. The "i-Real" was developed for the urban environment, tailored toward the transportation of a single adult. The device itself is compact and its size is roughly equivalent to that of a grown adult. The position and orientation of the seat promotes the togetherness of the driver and the vehicle. The

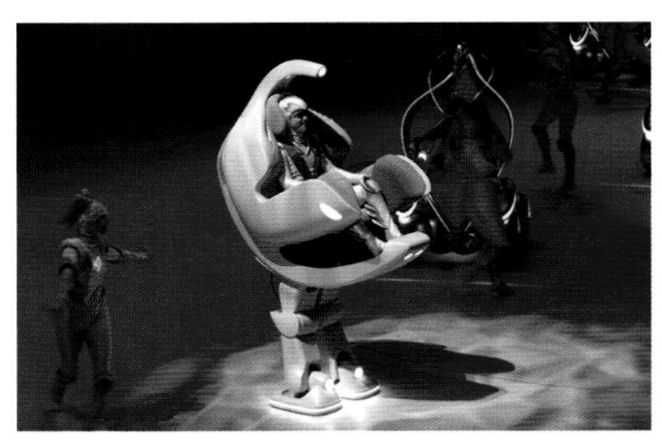
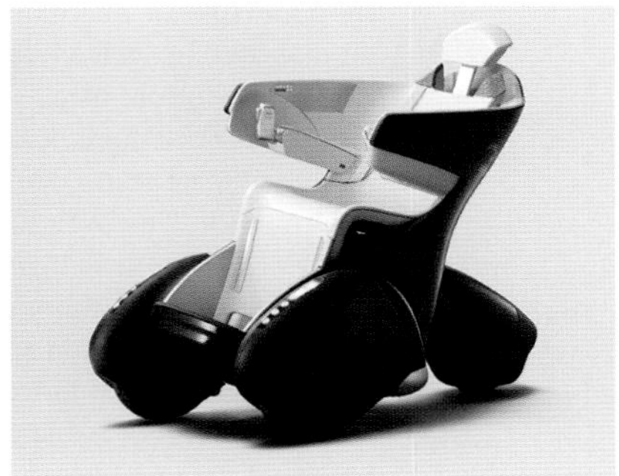

Figure 4.12 Left: i-foot.
Right: i-Real.
Source: Toyota

control of the "i-Real" is intuitive and done through fields of sensors implemented in the vehicle's armrests.

Technology: The "i-Real" is driven by an electromotor that drives both front tires. Its battery can be recharged via a standard electricity plug and the vehicle can travel for approximately 30 km on a single charge. With two optimized gears, the "i-Real" is a technical masterpiece. The vehicle is versatile as it can safely operate in pedestrian zones with a cruising speed of 6 km/h but also keep up with downtown traffic at a speed of 30 km/h. Depending on its use (and consequent intended speed), the position of the vehicle' wheels can vary. In the slower mode, the back tire is pulled in and the vehicle travels in a more upright position. In this way, the driver is more at "eyelevel" with other pedestrians. For the security of the driver and nearby pedestrians, the "i-Real" is constantly monitoring its immediate environment and warns the driver of possible collisions using both audio and optical warnings. In the fast mode, the back tire is pushed further out and the center of gravity of the vehicle is lowered, allowing the driver to sit in a more ergonomically position. Source: www.toyota.co.jp/en.

System Name: i-Swing
Developer: Toyota
The "i-Swing" (see Figure 4.13) follows other pod-like single-user transportation vehicles from Toyota and is their fourth instalment in developments of this nature. With its compact and flexible body, the "i-Swing" perfectly adapts to its individual use space. The "i-Swing" can be adjusted to fit the user's personal needs and provide them with nearly unlimited mobility. The "i-Swing" is actually equipped with two operating systems: one geared toward slower and more sensitive environments and the other for faster paced environments. For the first use environment, the system uses two-wheel drive that is very dependable and safe and allows for accurate control and navigation through pedestrian zones. For the second use environment, the system takes advantage of its three-wheel drive in order to provide high performance and agility in regular street traffic. With its multiple ultramodern communication functions, the "i-Swing" mobility concept goes far beyond the possibilities of conventional vehicles.

Technology: The form of the "i-Swing" does not resemble that of a traditional vehicle so much as it almost suggests a new lifeform. Its futuristic and minimalistic body is comprised of anti-shock polyurethane. Through its integrated intelligence system, the "i-Swing" can also remain in constant communication with its driver, even appearing like a virtual person on a

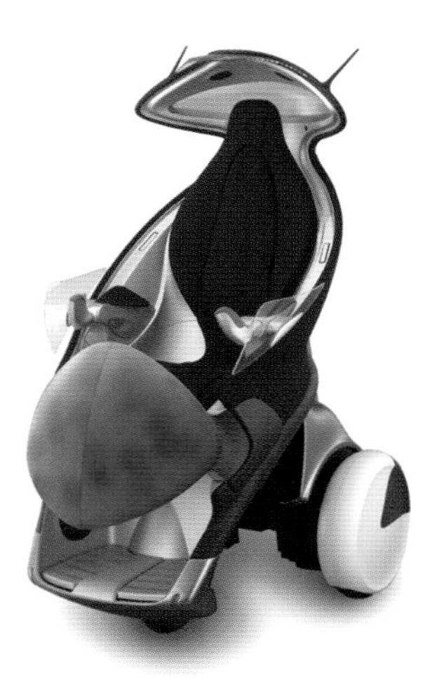

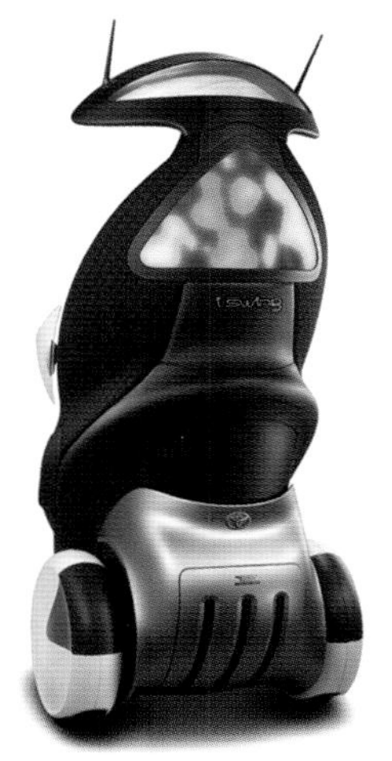

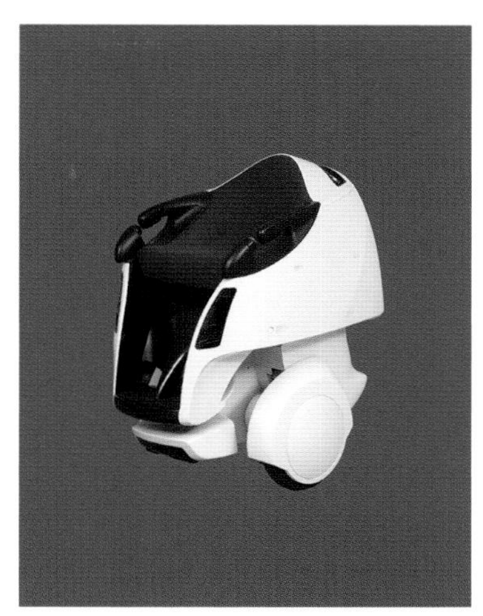

Figure 4.13 Left: i-Swing.
Right: Wheelchair Robot.
Source: Toyota

pop-up display at times. Over time, the vehicle learns the behavioral mannerisms of the driver and with this knowledge, can produce desired information and make adjustments accordingly. The material enclosure of the outer portion of the vehicle is interchangeable, allowing for users to put their personal touch on their vehicle. The front door and rear triangular portion of the vehicle are equipped with color LED matrices that allow displays of pictures, messages, or short videos, depending on the user's wish. Source: www.toyota.co.jp/en.

System Name: Wheelchair Robot
Developer: Toyota
The concept for the "Wheelchair Robot" (see Figure 4.13) from Toyota is to enable a comfortable way for users to travel short distances. The device is not only intended for transportation between one's workplace and home, but also for traveling distances within the workplace or within the home. This unit combines individual autonomous mobility with transport ability to replace the requirement of using one's own legs when getting around. Additionally, the "Wheelchair Robot" has a number of accessory functions. One such function is the ability for the unit to travel adjacent to its "user" and be used as a type of wagon to transport items with heavy loads.
Technology: The underlying concept of the "Wheelchair Robot" is that it is very compact and light compared with other units of similar function. This allows the unit to be easily transported and used across various locations. The device stands at only about 1 m high and this height is increased to only 1.1 m when compacted for transport. It weighs about 150 kg. The device can travel up to a speed of 6.0 km/h and can last for approximately 20 km on a single charge. Source: www.toyota.co.jp/en.

System Name: RCAST Group: Space Technology for Rehabilitation Science
Developer: JAXA Institute
The JAXA Institute is attempting to transfer their technical knowhow in the spaceflight industry into the field of nursing care. As they are among those that best understand the need for lightweight construction material and kinematics, they hope to use this knowledge to

develop a solution that reduces the strain of heavy lifting often required by nursing staff. The use of a GPS controlled wheelchair with an integrated navigation system as well as the use of a special matrix display for the blind are just a few examples of the effectiveness of their approach.

Technology: Due to the strains of heavy lifting, lightweight equipment, materials, and kinematics are especially important in the field of nursing and caregiving. This transportation system was developed specifically for this domain. The system enables the transportation of patients from one bed to another without large efforts from staff. The specially developed Braille display enables blind users to control and steer the system. The display functions similarly to conventional touch panels but instead of two-dimensional graphics, it is equipped with the ability to produce surfaces that can be touched and understood by those unable to see them. The specially constructed lightweight wheelchair ("Dream Carry") is comprised mostly of modern plastics and synthetic materials. This allows it to maintain a weight of only 5.5 kg. The chair can also be folded into two half-suitcase shells and be transported by simply carrying around the suitcase. This allows for easy and comfortable transportation to almost anywhere. Source: RCAST Group, Prof. S. Fukushima, Tokyo University, JAXA Japan Aerospace Exploration Agency.

System Name: i-Road (Personal Mobility)
Developer: Toyota
Driving through Japanese metropolitan areas becomes problematic with the high prices for parking spots and the inability to even find such spots in the first place. Without parking spaces, the option of driving becomes impractical. Special exceptions have been made by the Japanese government for tiny city vehicles or "Kei-Cars". As such, the demand for these tiny two-seated vehicles has drastically increased. Toyota unveiled the i-Road (or PersonalMobility, PM, see Figure 4.14) at the Tokyo motor show to address this increase in demand for "Kei-Cars". The vehicle is enclosed with an egg-like shell that fits snugly around the single user. Toyota goes so far as to call their 1.75 m tall i-Road "the first wearable vehicle in the world".

Technology: The rolling egg-shaped i-Real is able to change its shape based on its specific use case. The driver cabin remains upright or tilts downward depending on where the vehicle is

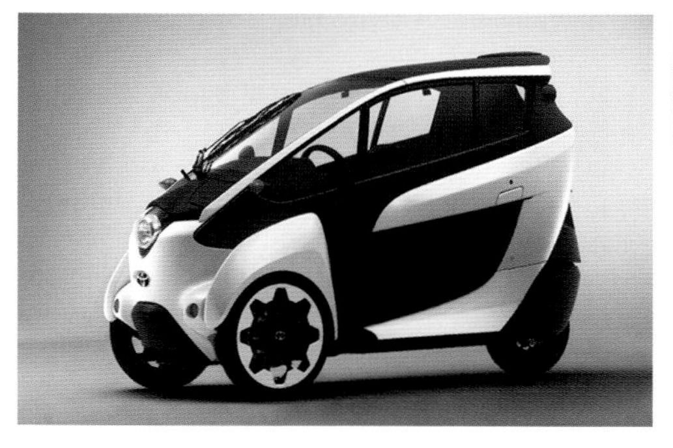

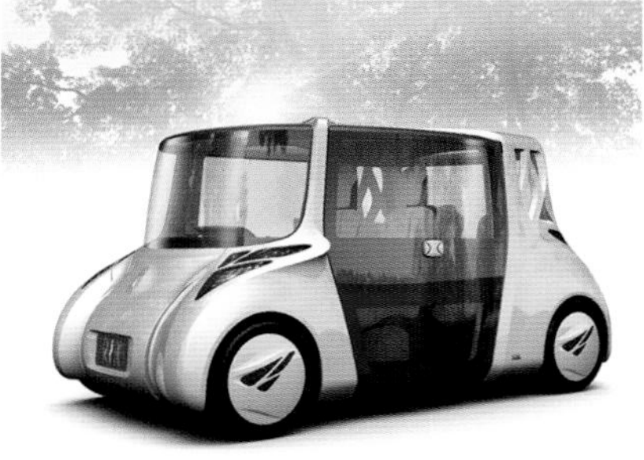

Figure 4.14 Left: i-Road.
Right: Toyota RIN Interior.
Source: Toyota

being driven. In slower, city traffic, the cabin remains upright and provides the user a good view of their entire surroundings. During faster highway use, the cabin reclines in order to become more aerodynamic. For entering and exiting the vehicle, the cabin is in the upright position to allow the user easy access and comfortable transitions. The entire front door also opens upwards to enable unhindered access. After the door opens, the seat moves outwards to allow easier entering of the vehicle. Steering of the vehicle is controlled by two joysticks adjacent to the seat. Only the front wheels are used for steering and actually pivot to allow turning on the spot. The i-Road is also able to identify and communicate with other i-Real vehicles, even changing its color as it does so. This feature also enables the vehicles to form a sort of marching line where one vehicle is in charge of leading, and the other simply follow in an auto piloted manner. Source: www.toyota.co.jp/en.

System Name: Toyota Mobility Assistance Program
Developer: Toyota
The motivation behind this recently developed approach is the notion that senior and/or disabled people should not be discriminated against in Japan. With this goal in mind, Toyota is seeking to offer specific individual transportation solutions based on the disabilities of customers. Their product portfolio ranges from simple machines such as a hand crank to fully automated wheel chair integration into vehicles. With this approach, they hope to respect the different vehicle categories (and often, financial backgrounds) that are present among various customers. The themes of "Universal Design" and "Mass Customization" are present in all technical requirements of the various products available.
Technology: The "Transport Wheelchair" (visible in Figure 4.14) allows users the possibility to enter and exit a vehicle without the need for lifting themselves from their chair. While the user remains seated, the undercarriage of the wheelchair is pushed over rails and loaded onto an adjustable seat. The tillable and adjustable seat is very advantageous for those with problems when entering and exiting vehicles. The seat is able to be maneuvered outside the limits of the vehicle in order to provide easy access. The seat is adjustable in both height and angle to allow the "sideways" loading of users from wheelchairs. The pivoting of the seat can be controlled either manually or automatically and the lowering or raising of the seat is accomplished with the help of an electric motor. A wireless remote control is optional. The final position of the seat is programmable for ease of repeated use. Source: www.toyota.co.jp/en.

System Name: Toyota RIN Interior
Developer: Toyota
The gently opening sliding doors of the Toyota RIN Interior (see Figure 4.14) remind one of the doors of a Japanese teahouse. The goal of its development was for the driver to feel a sense of relaxation as if they were actually entering the said teahouse. The warmth of the heated seat, the posture in which it encourages, and its upright position are also used to resemble those of the traditional Japanese tea ceremony. In fact, the term mediation is even found in its name, RiN, representative of the Chinese characters for "upright position". For both the interior and exterior of the vehicle, developers were inspired by the Yakusugi Tree, a Japanese Cyprus. This was intended to keep users in tune with nature and to establish a healthy balance between body and soul. To continue with the focus on environment, an oxygen regulator and air humidifier help the vehicle to maintain an optimal temperature, oxygen level, and humidity level.
Technology: The RiN abstains from the classical steering wheel in favor of a steering control resembling that of an airplane. The vehicle is also equipped with a series of sensors that record vital signs data in a similar way as an electrocardiogram (ECG). The dashboard also features a screen that displays images that are intended to influence the mood of the driver in a

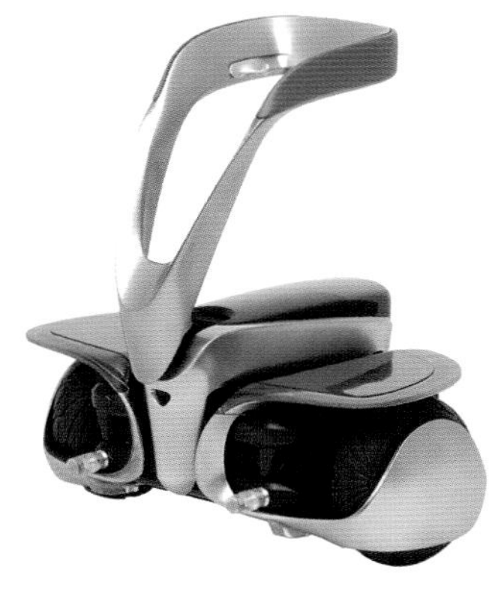

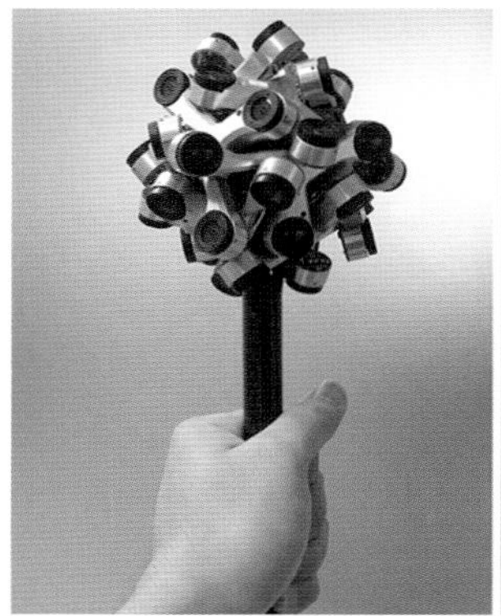

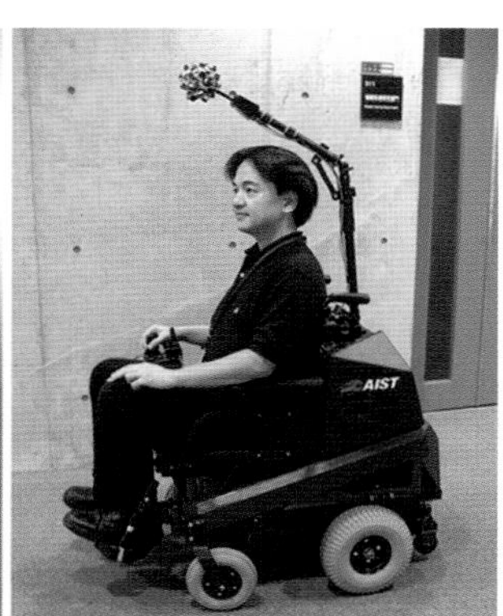

Figure 4.15 Left: Toyota WINGLET.
Source: Toyota
Right: AIST Intelligent Wheelchair.
Source: Yutaka Satoh, AIST

positive manner. These gentle changes of images subconsciously relax the user. The green tinted glass windshield of the vehicle decreases the penetration of harmful UV rays while allowing lots of natural light into the vehicle. The lower windows and doors of the vehicle are also transparent in order to improve the driver's overall view of their surroundings. The 3.25 m long, 1.69 m wide, and 1.65 m high RiN is also considerate of other drivers on the road. The vehicle has a special function that allows the strategic distribution of light from the headlights away from oncoming traffic in order to temporarily avoid blinding them. Source: www.toyota.co.jp/en.

System Name: Toyota Sustainable Mobility WINGLET
Developer: Toyota
The futuristic Toyota WINGLET (see Figure 4.15) requires no special driving abilities from its users. It remains balanced between its two wheels and is useful in everyday situations. The vehicle is compact, yet strong, and can be charged from any conventional electrical outlet. It presents new opportunities in business life as workers can expand their mobility, sense of their surroundings, and load carrying capacity. The WINGLET accomplishes these functions through a variety of modern technologies. The machine is intended to be used at Japanese airports and will later be tested in large urban centers and shopping malls in order to gauge reactions from various users.
Technology: The Toyota WINGLET is available in three different versions, however, the platform of the vehicle is constant across all three versions. The difference appears in the height of the vehicle shaft. The Model L has a shaft that reaches approximately waist high or 1.13 m, the Model M to the knee or 0.68 m, and the Model S to the calf or 0.46 m. The two larger versions weigh approximately 12.3 kg with the smaller Model S weighing in at just 10 kg. The different versions are intended to accommodate different use cases. Toyota deems the vehicle suitable for users from "practical to those attempting to ride hands free for excitement". The maximum speed of the vehicle is about 6 km/h, yet the vehicle boasts a turning radius of 0 m allowing it to be very agile. The maximum range of the vehicle is between 5 and 10 kms depending on the use case, and recharging is completed in just one hour. Source: www.toyota.co.jp/en.

System Name: AIST Intelligent Wheelchair
Developer: AIST, Yutaka Satoh
The development of the AIST Intelligent Wheelchair (visible in Figure 4.15) is aimed at enhancing the quality of life for older people with higher needs in terms of their social environment. This technology offers those that are bound to a wheelchair the opportunity to move more independently. Due to this increased assistance with mobility, there is also an increase in potential dangers for the user in terms of accidents with other drivers. For this reason, this robot was developed in order to monitor the surroundings of the user and avoid these risks.
Technology: The AIST features a stereo omnidirectional system (developed by Yataka Satoh in the JST Human and Object Interaction Processing Project) that is able to produce, in real time, moving colorful images with the help of 36 mounted cameras. The system uses this to create a 3-dimensional model of its immediate surroundings. The cameras are organized in such a way that there are no blind spots when using this technology. The logical positioning of the system over the wheelchair provides it with the best possible location to accurately and efficiently capture all of its surroundings. With this information, the wheelchair is able to pre-emptively brake in the event that it senses danger or possible collisions. Source: www.aist.go.jp/index_en.html.

System Name: Suzuki SSC
Developer: Suzuki
The Suzuki SSC (Suzuki Sharing Coach, shown in Figure 4.16) is a "minicar-based mobility unit" intended to be paired with the Suzuki PIXY. The PIXY is a single-user pod-like scooter based on the concept of "friendly mobility". It is intended for low speed operation on pedestrian footpaths and inside of buildings. The SSC is paired with the PIXY in order to form a more traditional looking automobile for higher speed operation among regular street traffic. One SSC is capable of holding a maximum of two PIXY vehicles. The PIXY can also be coupled with a sports-car version (SSF) and a boat unit (SSJ). The project aims at achieving a sustainable mobility system in accordance with the Japanese Ministry of

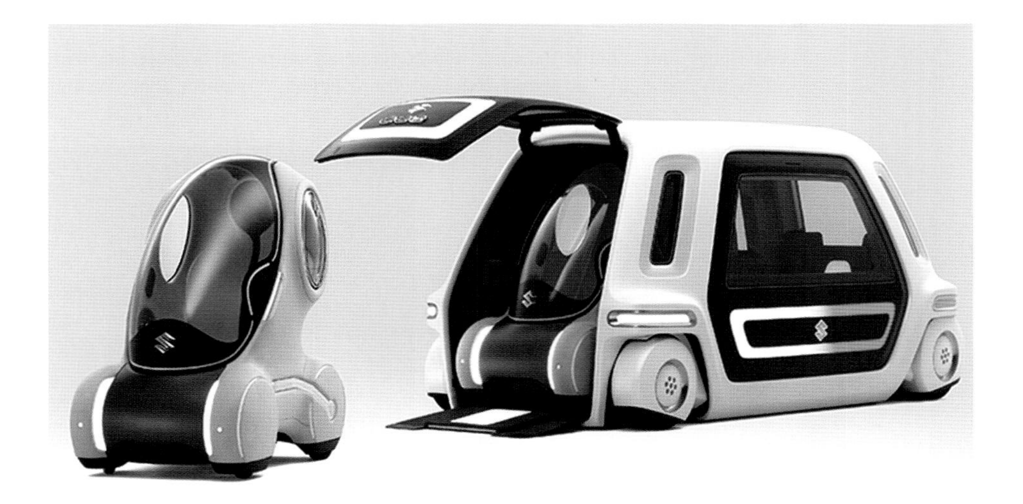

Figure 4.16 Suzuki SSC.
Source: Suzuki

Economy and Trade as well as the Industry's Next Generation Vehicle and Fuel initiative, aimed at realizing an environmentally friendly "people-centred motorized society." Source: www.suzuki.co.jp/.

System Name: Universal Vehicle RODEM
Developer: TMSUK Co.
The "universal vehicle" was developed with the elderly and physically disabled in mind as it was designed in such a way that users can enter and exit the vehicle with ease due to limited constraints. This allows for use of the vehicle without the need for care staff to assist in the boarding or alighting of the vehicle. It is equipped with many special features and aims at providing users with an opportunity to freely travel wherever they want to go.
Technology: The "Universal Vehicle RODEM" is also equipped with some special features. It has a built-in GPS navigation system for traversing through unknown parts of the city. It is also equipped with an automatic obstacle evasion mechanism to avoid collisions. An automatic slope correction system, autonomous navigation function, and voice recognition also assist in its use. The vehicle also features a vital sign monitoring system, a feature especially valuable for senior users. The vehicle is 1220 x 690 x 1170 mm in size. It requires a charging time of approximately 4 hours and has a maximum speed of 6.0 km/h. Source: www.tmsuk.co.jp/en/.

System Name: City-Car PIVO
Developer: Nissan, Takashi Murakimi, Cyberdyne, Tsukuba University
The PIVO is a futuristic concept car from Nissan and is characterized by its unique pivoting cabin. The car is fully electric and features excellent visibility from all sides of the vehicle. This visibility is further enhanced by Nissan's "Around View" technology, eliminating various blind spots around the car. The car is also very compact and easy to maneuver. In addition to the pivoting cabin, the second iteration of the PIVO also features pivoting wheels. This provides drivers with much more flexibility and makes parallel parking, and even reversing altogether, a thing of the past. As the wheels can pivot 90 degrees, users can simply drive sideways in and out of a tight parking spot. Despite an overall length of only 2.7 m, the car comfortably fits three passengers and is easy to get into and out of thanks to its tall, power sliding doors.
Technology: The cabin of the car is able to rotate an entire 360 degrees, allowing the driver to comfortably face any direction required for efficient operation. For example, instead of

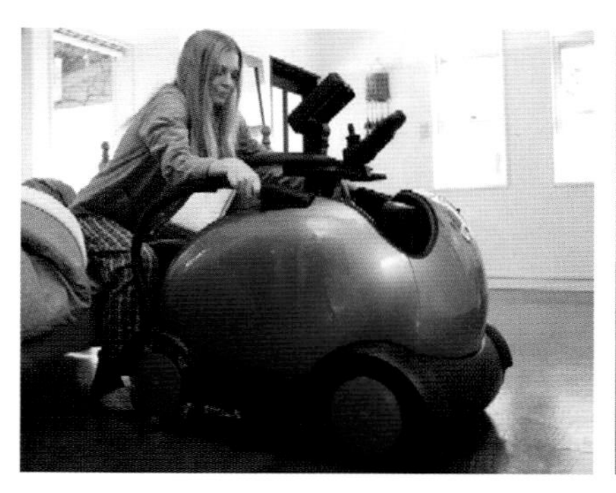

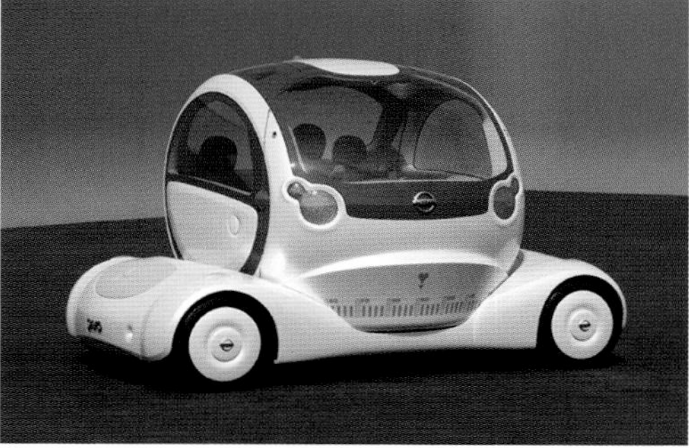

Figure 4.17 Left: Universal Vehicle RODEM.
Source: TMSUK
Right: City-Car PIVO.
Source: Nissan

reversing, the driver can simply rotate the cabin and drive "forwards" in the opposite direction. The pivoting function of the wheels is powered by an in-wheel electric motor for each individual wheel, with the charge coming from lithium-ion batteries. The PIVO is itself powered by Nissan's unique Supermotor, which results in zero emissions. Each axel is powered by its own Supermotor, allowing them to be controlled independently for an even distribution of torque to all four wheels. Nissan's unique "Drive by Wire" technologies allow control of various functions of the car to occur electronically, rather than the conventional mechanical method. In addition to the rotation of the cabin, the "Drive by Wire" approach allows electronic control of the steering, braking, shifting, and signaling. This approach removes the need for mechanical linkages between the cabin and the undercarriage, thus enabling the possibility of a rotating cabin. The PIVO is also equipped with a robotic agent that assists in navigation, control of various features in the car, and even finding nearby parking spaces. Source: www.cyberdyne.jp; www.elm-design.com.

5 Research and Development Projects for AAL Systems

In this chapter, several projects will be presented in order to show the current state of the art in the research and development of the integration of ambient integrated robotics. The projects focus especially on the support of the elderly and fragile people. The main aim of each single project is to keep the user physically and mentally active in order to slow down the process of senility. All the tasks that the user cannot do alone anymore must be supported by the technology. Here however, the main difficulty in each presented project is to establish the system in a way that only the minimal necessary support is offered, otherwise the user could become too inactive leading to an accelerated process of senility.

5.1 Project GEWOS

The objective of GEWOS (Gesund wohnen mit Stil – Healthy Living with Style) was to develop a sociotechnical furniture that animates the elderly to move more actively, in order to enable a healthy lifestyle. By implementing the appropriate technology into an armchair for the living room, this health-support system is unobtrusively integrated into the living environment of the elderly. The overall system consists of motion sensor unobtrusively integrated into the seat, training devices (e.g., rows), a TV (as interface), and some vital measurement devices like pulse oximetry and ECG. By using Wi-Fi, the armchair measurement gets directly connected with a server (via internet). Using a remote controller concludes the overall system integration into a smart living environment, allowing to not only control the TV and display measurement results, but also to control home electronics like light switches.

A specially designed graphical user interface (GUI) allows the elderly an intuitive access to the different service functions offered by the chair. However, the project confirmed the importance of the end-user motivation and design if such systems should be applied in the user's home environment. In order to enable training and at the same time make the armchair look convenient, rowing oars have been integrated into the chair. The oars are covered by the arm rest, which let the armchair look like a normal armchair. Stand-assist as well as position is also provided, which allows the user to train (guided by the GUI of the GEWOS TV) directly on the chair (see Figure 5.2).

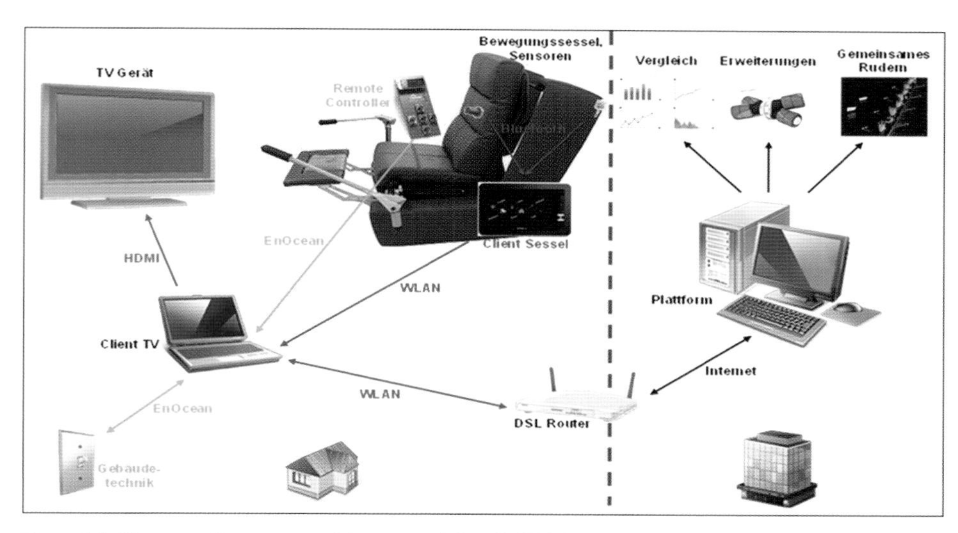

Figure 5.1 The overall system architecture of the GEWOS project.

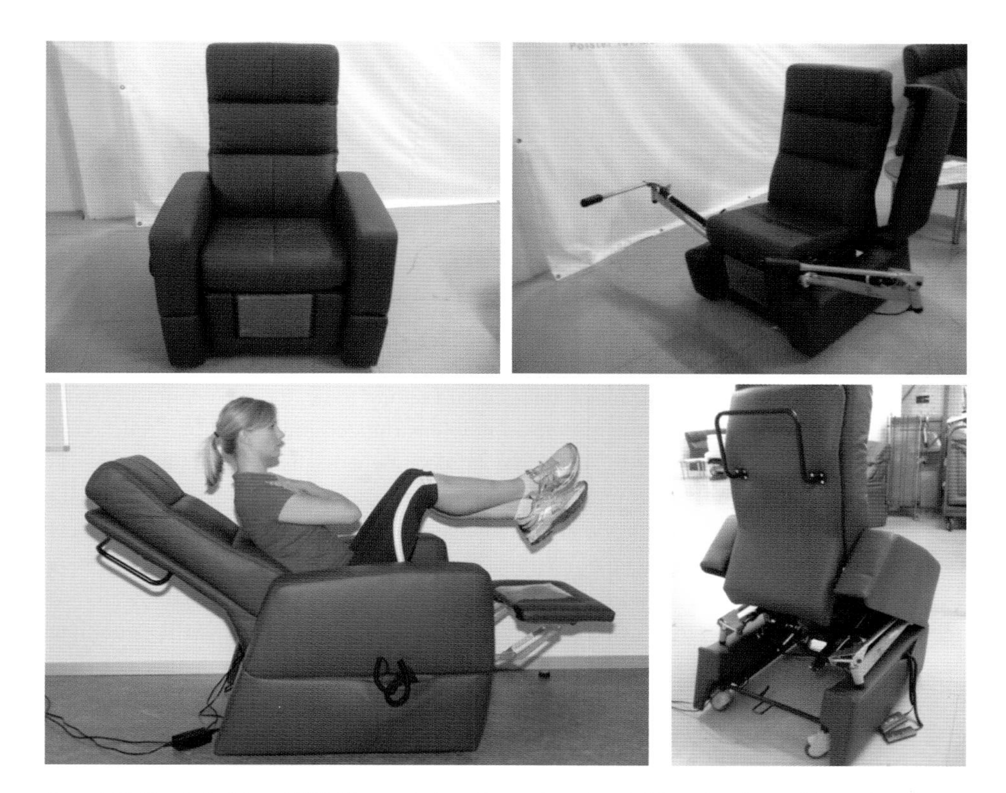

Figure 5.2 Top left: The GEWOS armchair with unobtrusive AAL technology. Top right: The GEWOS armchair with uncovered rows. Bottom left: Stand-assist. Bottom right: Training guided by the GEWOS GUI.

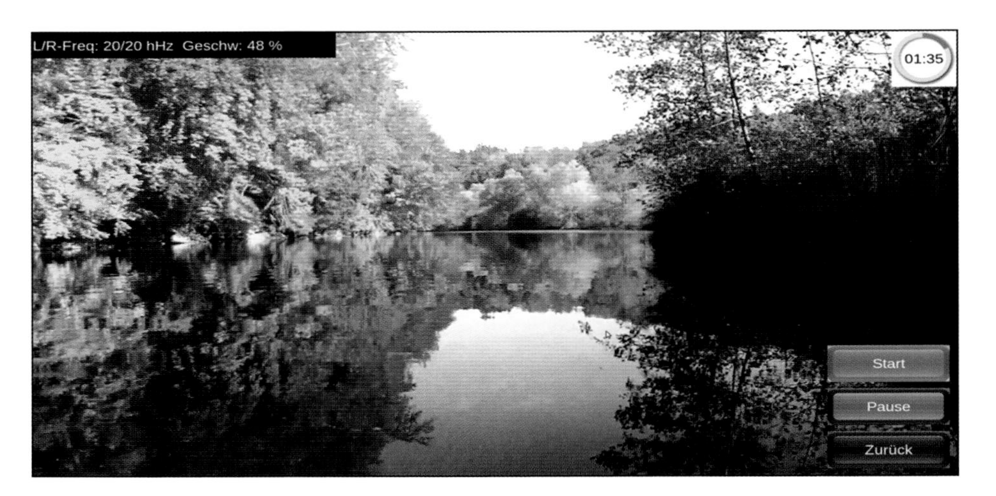

Figure 5.3 Virtual river trip for training guided movements.

To motivate the user to train, a video-gaming style has been implemented. As Figure 5.3 demonstrates, the user sees a virtual river, which he can row down, using the implemented oars in the arm rests. While the elderly is just playing a game, he is in fact training guided movements via use of the oars.

5.2 Project LISA

Devices, like those mentioned in Section 5.1, can be expensive to replace an existing furniture. Although this fact does not sound so critical, the elderly do not easily separate from their belongings, because they link them with memories. Therefore, for the AAL research, it is a major topic to develop add-ons, which are also compatible with the given environment.

This is one of the most challenging factors: to develop a technology that can be easily installed in a different and absolutely customized, but not structured, user environment. For example, a more structured environment is the car. If someone wants to install a navigation device into a car, the installation is easier, because of the standardization (in this case the windscreen). In an apartment, this luxury does not exist; even door sizes differ from apartment to apartment. Nevertheless, project LISA's objective is to find a solution here by developing plug-and-play smart AAL walls. Additionally, the multimorbidity of the elderly must be considered, which leads to complex and highly individual multiple constraints. Therefore, the multidimensionality, i.e., the possibility to operate several modules of the offered assistance at once is of central importance [157].

For the very first time, the apartment was structured in their different areas: living room, bed room, kitchen, bath room, and entrance areas (see Figure 5.4).

For each area, a unique solution must be found. To do this, a basic module, which can easily be installed (in a few hours) must be developed. This smart wall device will later on serve as an interface for various modules that offer different services.

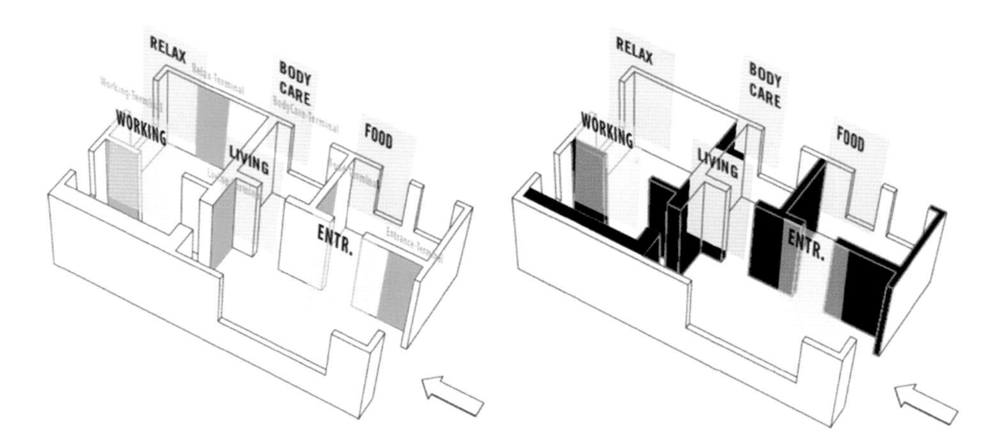

Figure 5.4 Identified apartment areas and the estimation regarding the free space on the walls.

Depending on the apartment area, the offered services must distinguish that, e.g., an induction cooker is very useful in the kitchen but makes less sense in the entrance area. According to this new approach, the different apartment areas have been evaluated according to their interface complexity (current, internet, water supply, etc.). The results showed that the entrance area belongs to the most promising areas, according to the high need of the elderly (here the elderly and fragile face a lot of challenges, forgetting keys or choosing the wrong coat for the actual weather condition, which may lead to influenza, etc.) and the least complexity regarding the interface compared to the bathroom and kitchen, which need a water supply interface.

As the next necessary step in this approach, the service functions must be defined. According to the project, investigations following overall functions have been considered (also illustrated in Figure 5.9): light (including color and intensity), remembering function (to avoid that the elderly lose or forget their keys, etc.), shoehorn (to ease dressing), vital measurements (to figure out potential risks of diseases together with the weather report), robotic assistance (to carry the belongings of the user), and a stand-assist (for the case of a weak blood circulation).

There are some functions already on the market, like the vital measurement, which has been implemented in the terminal. Every household has a blood pressure meter, a scale, or a blood glucose meter. Here, however, the main objective of the project LISA is the seamless integration or interfacing of these existing products. The mentioned devices use a Wi-Fi transmission to send their data to a local server, which is used to store the data, in order to plot them on a user-friendly GUI and to show the health status over time. This allows to more efficiently interpret, e.g., blood pressure, as the measurements work in relation to each other instead of just giving a single result. The overall system architecture is depicted in Figure 5.6, and also shows the communication to the reminding function.

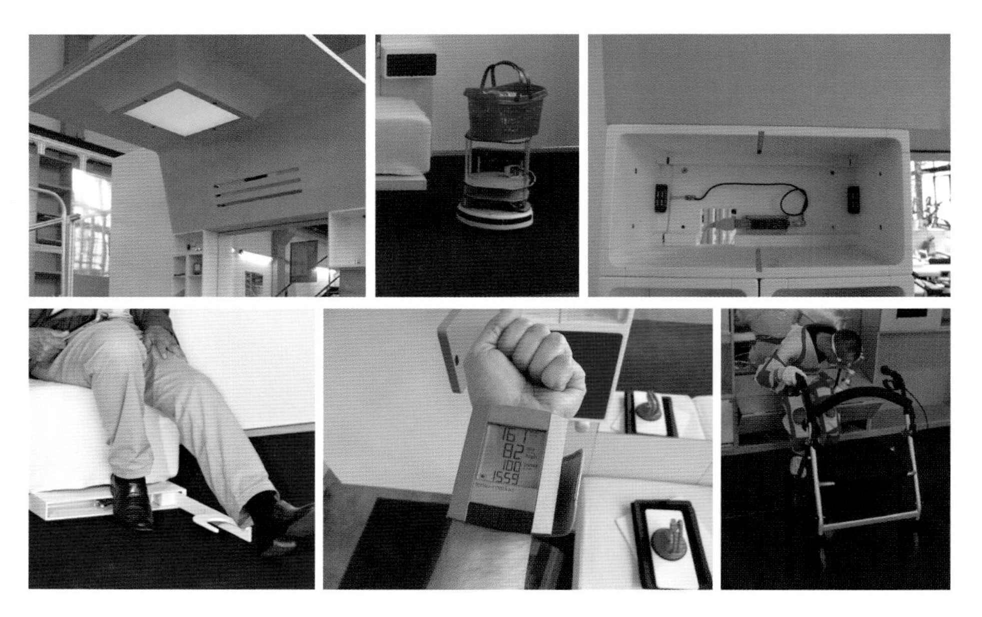

Figure 5.5 Potential service modules for the smart AAL walls. Top left: Light and air purifier. Top middle: Robotic assistance. Top right: RFID Antenna and processing unit with USB interface. Bottom left: Shoehorn for dressing assistance. Bottom middle: Blood pressure meter for health status estimation. Bottom right: Stand-assist.

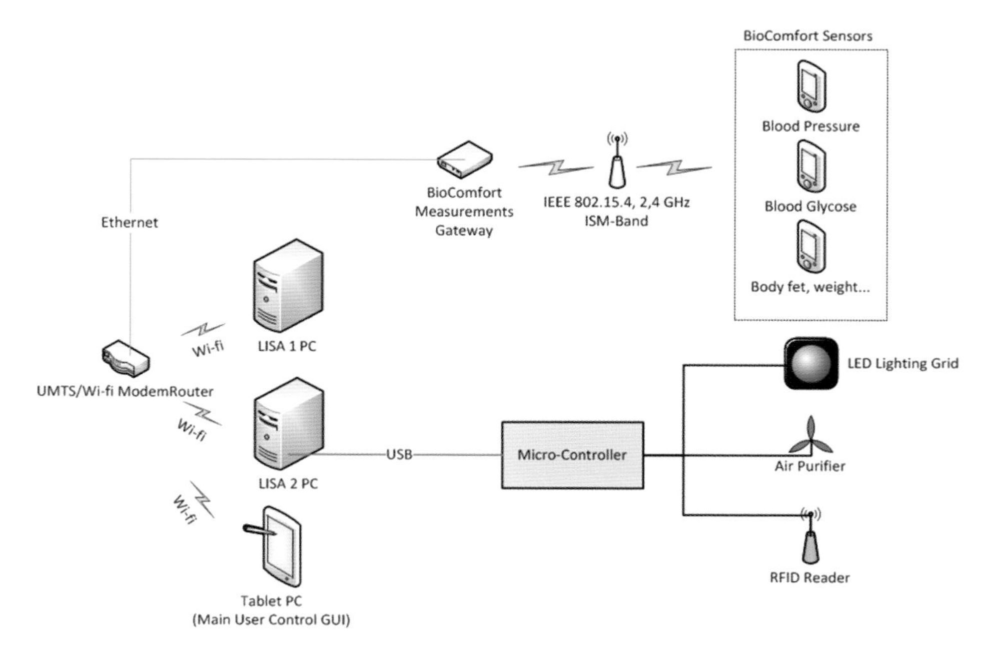

Figure 5.6 Overall system architecture of the smart LISA AAL wall.

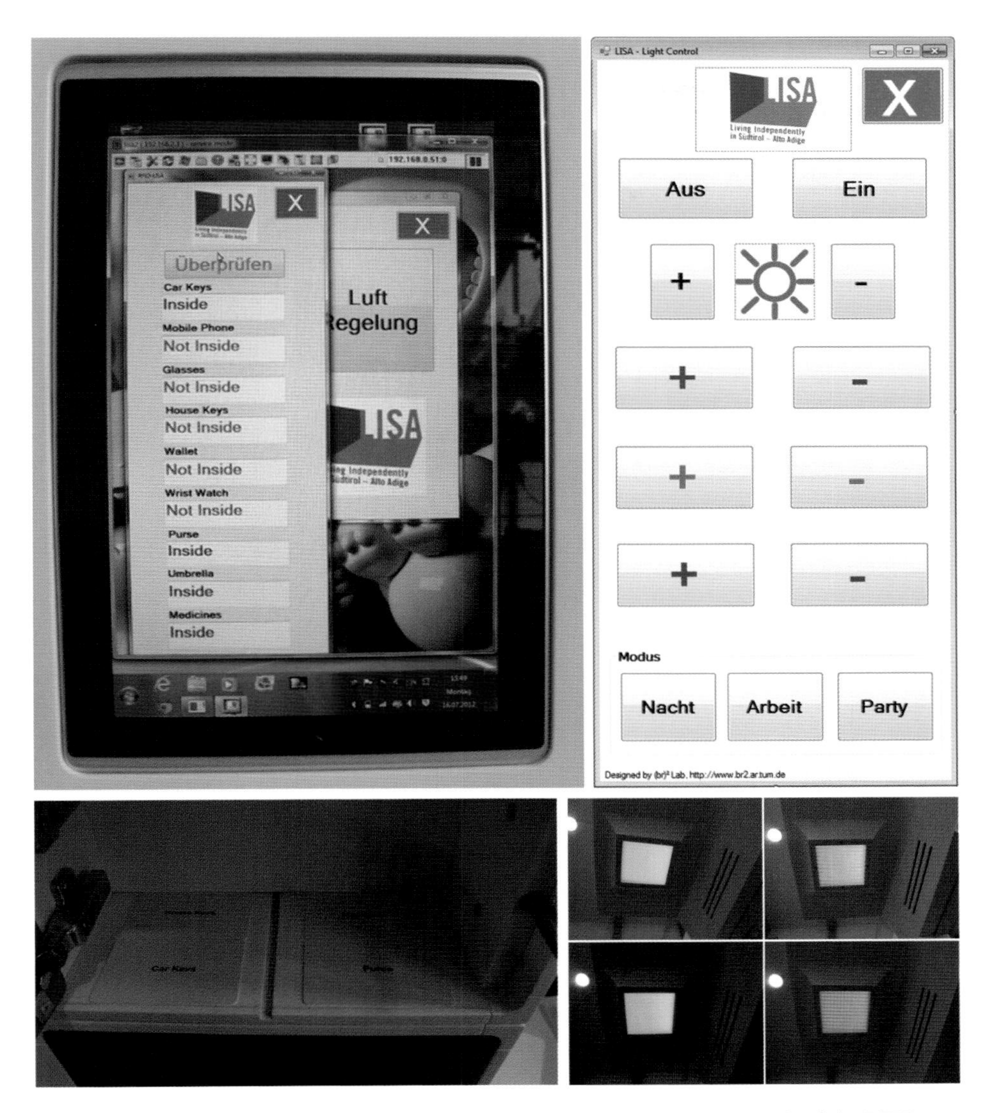

Figure 5.7 Top left: GUI on the touch screen as user interface, showing the result of the RFID tag scan. Bottom left: The test tags in the shelf for demonstration. Top right: An exemplary user interface for setting up the light condition. Bottom right: The different results which can be set up.

The reminding function uses RFID technology to identify, by tags, the appropriately marked objects. The tags are passively powered and can be very small, which allows for marking, e.g., the keys unobtrusively. An antenna implemented in each shell of the shelf is able to detect the tag (see Figure 5.5). Using Arduino Micro as the processing unit, it is possible to read out the RFID antenna and to forward the information to the local server, where the availability information of the object is stored. The user can access the information by using the LISA GUI as shown in Figure 5.7. As the Arduino is supplied and interfaced by USB, this

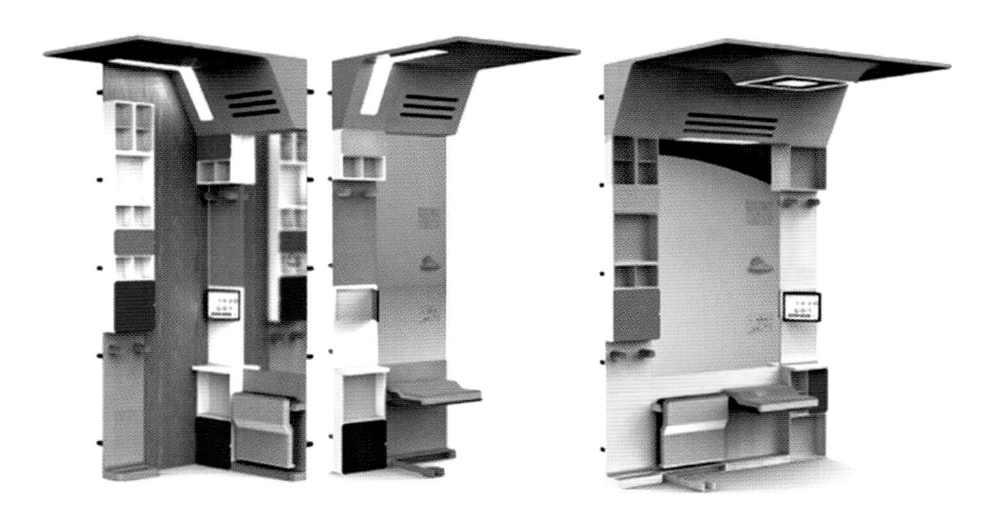

Figure 5.8 Different setting of the smart AAL wall LISA. Left: the light version. Right: the full version.

function is easy to install by plug-and-play, which means that the modularity aspect is fulfilled.

The GUI allows the user to also control the function of the light and air conditioner [158]. It also showed that the light color and intensity can directly influence the mood of a senior. Additionally, the potential is given to link the RFID remind function to the light, e.g., when the door is opened, in order to enable a silent (i.e., not stigmatizing) alert, which warns the user not to forget the key in the shelf, before closing the door.

The modularity aspect of the smart AAL wall LISA is not limited to the potential service modules. As part of customization, and considering the different sizes of the apartments, the terminals can be set up as shown in Figure 5.8.

5.3 Project PASSAge

Mobility means life quality, especially in old age. Therefore, it is not surprising that there exists a huge variety of mobility aids (rollator, Stairlift, E-Scooters, etc.). Up to now, however, it is still very challenging for the elderly to take part in the public road traffic. This is mostly because when mobility aids are being developed (or houses, trains, etc.), the interface for these aids are mostly neglected. For example, the rollator is nowadays helping a lot of the elderly to stay mobile. However, there are a lot of entrance doors, which have "just" three steps (because it looks nice). Unfortunately, for someone who is fragile and needs a rollator as support, the three steps are invincible with the rollator.

Here, the PASSAge project aimed to investigate such "mobility gaps" in order to design interfaces on the hard- and software level to develop a seamless mobility chain from the bed to the entire world. The major focus in this section will be on the home environment.

Demographic changes have an impact on the future planning of the mobility for an independent life. Accessibility, according to the existing standards, can only partially solve the problem; therefore, holistic concepts are needed. Distances, which can be done by foot or by bicycle are usually straightforward, but the risk for elderly as pedestrians or cyclists is high. For example, as pedestrians, the risk to die by an accident is increased by 3.8 times. On the other hand, the risk of cyclists getting killed by an accident increases by 5.8 times according to [159].

This is because of age-related reduction of the physical and cognitive competencies among the elderly, which can lead to small mistakes with serious consequences. To secure the mobility of the elderly, existing mobility aids like the rollator should be further developed by add-ons, and additionally taking into account that future seniors will be healthier and more mobile than the current elderly [160]. The objective of the project was to provide a cross-linked and flexible infrastructure for a variety of mobility components, where the different components are not in competition with each other but create synergies by cooperation in order to secure the mobility and agility of the elderly. The smartphone is thought to be an interface for controlling the PASSAge System environment, which could also be used for navigation and health management (using appropriate apps).

Different constellations and connections in the value system offering different optimal solutions are what institutions and companies concentrate on in the development of assistance and aid systems [161]. Four different scenarios (or use cases) were defined in order to estimate the potentially best solutions within PASSAge. The first use case is the AAL-House, including care phones, safety bracelets, video telephony, alarm detectors for smoke water, etc. The second use case considered E-Cars of different sizes, walking aids, rollators, scooters, lift systems, and social services. The third use case described shopping, errands, doctors and hospital visits, culture and church events, visiting friends, and relatives. The fourth use case considered user interfaces, e.g., on smartphones, vital signs measurement (blood pressure, activity profile), navigation, service platforms, etc.

The main focus is set to Use Cases 1 and 2. Especially for the Use Case 1, the indoor support and use of robots has been investigated. Robots are difficult to include into the home environment, because they are mostly large, heavy, and expensive. Therefore, the use of the TurtleBot has been investigated.

The TurtleBot, for robots, is low-cost, lightweight, and small. Its disadvantage is the reduced payload, which leads to the question: how can a robot, which resembles a toy, support the elderly in their activities and mobility? For this purpose, a new interface (using PLE with a 3D printer), which allows the robot to connect to a rollator has been designed as demonstrated in Figure 5.9.

This approach allows the TurtleBot to move the rollator to the user, despite the payload being very low. The main idea behind this development is to ensure that an end

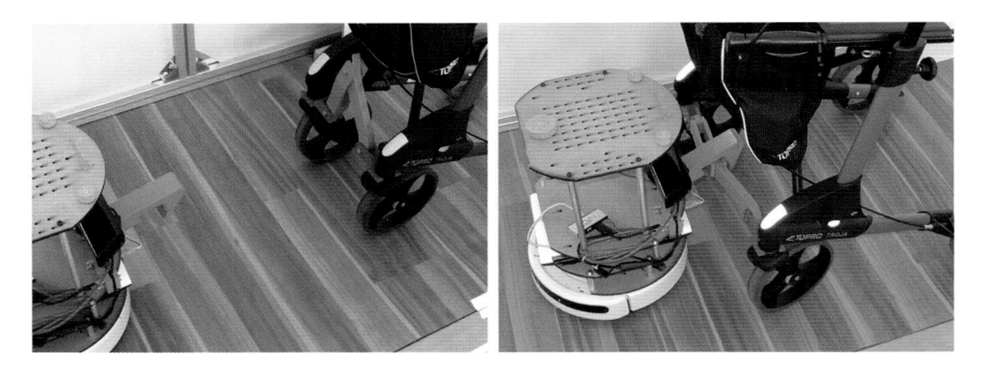

Figure 5.9 The new interface, which allows the TurtleBot to interface with the rollator.

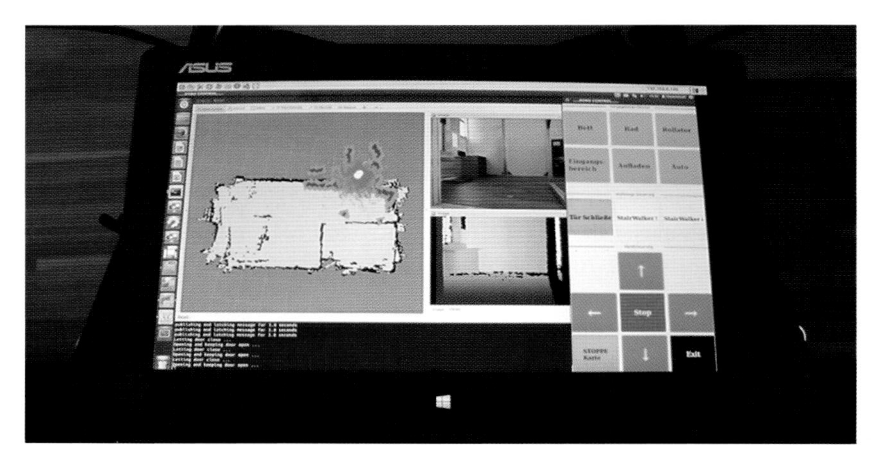

Figure 5.10 User interface, which allows the user to command and navigate the TurtleBot.

user can always reach the rollator by ultra-low-cost robots. However, this idea has the challenge to answer the question: how can a user control this robot?

To investigate the potentially best solution, a special GUI has been designed (shown in Figure 5.10), where the end user could test different controlling options.

The arrow buttons allow the user to directly navigate the robot. A map, showing the location of the robot in the apartment as well as the RGB image (and depth image), gives the user a hint as to where the robot is (in case the robot is hiding in another room). Even though this kind of control is very challenging for the elderly, it always offers the possibility to interfere if the robot is making a mistake.

At the top, predefined tasks, e.g., how to connect to a rollator, are defined. By pressing one of these buttons (using the touch screen of the tablet PC depicted in the window), the robot acts completely independent. Even though this kind of user input is preferred, the accuracy of the navigation of the TurtleBot is just enough to connect with the rollator. If the task needs a higher accuracy, the user must support the TurtleBot by the arrow buttons (Figure 5.1).

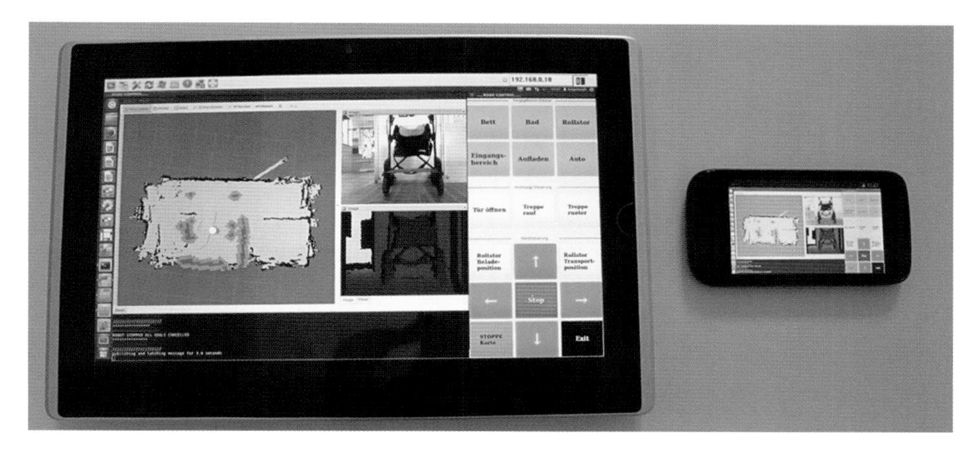

Figure 5.11 Left: A tablet PC with Windows 7 as the operating system. Right: A smartphone with Android as operating system.

Alternative inputs, like gesture control using the Leap motion sensor (as described in Section 5.4), or by voice control, showed a disappointing and weak result. The motion control is not intuitive enough for a mobile platform, whereas voice control fails mostly because of the different pronunciations, which are often influenced by dialects. Additionally, for the elderly, it is difficult to recall specific terms and to understand that they cannot talk to the robot like to a human, at least with current technology.

The alternative to pointing a position directly on the map by using the touchscreen was also not highly appreciated by the end user. However, still more preferred it to arrow buttons; the main critique of the touchscreen was that it is mostly too small to point to the correct position (especially on a smartphone, as shown in Figure 5.11). Combined with the reduced accuracy of the TurtleBot, the navigation of the robot becomes challenging again. Nevertheless, the subjects of the test mainly criticized the interface. As soon as the tester got used to the control option, the feedback was mainly good. This demonstrates the high potential of even such small and cheap robots like the TurtleBot.

The main challenge here is only to find an appropriate interface to control the necessary service task. According to [162], the use of smartphones or tablet PCs is an intuitive way to offer services to the elderly.

Because they lack haptic feedback, touchscreens are not the best solution. Voice control will become an optimal solution, if the matching algorithm becomes more robust. Autonomous and independent working robots demonstrated the highest user acceptance in the test.

Considering Use Case 2 of Figure 5.9, stairs are a major challenge for the TurtleBot as well as for rollator or wheelchair users. Therefore, transport options have been added to a device, which is named "StairWalker" (see Figure 5.12).

The StairWalker is comparable to a stair lift, with the difference being that there is no existing sitting place. This means that the user has to walk up and down the stairs on his

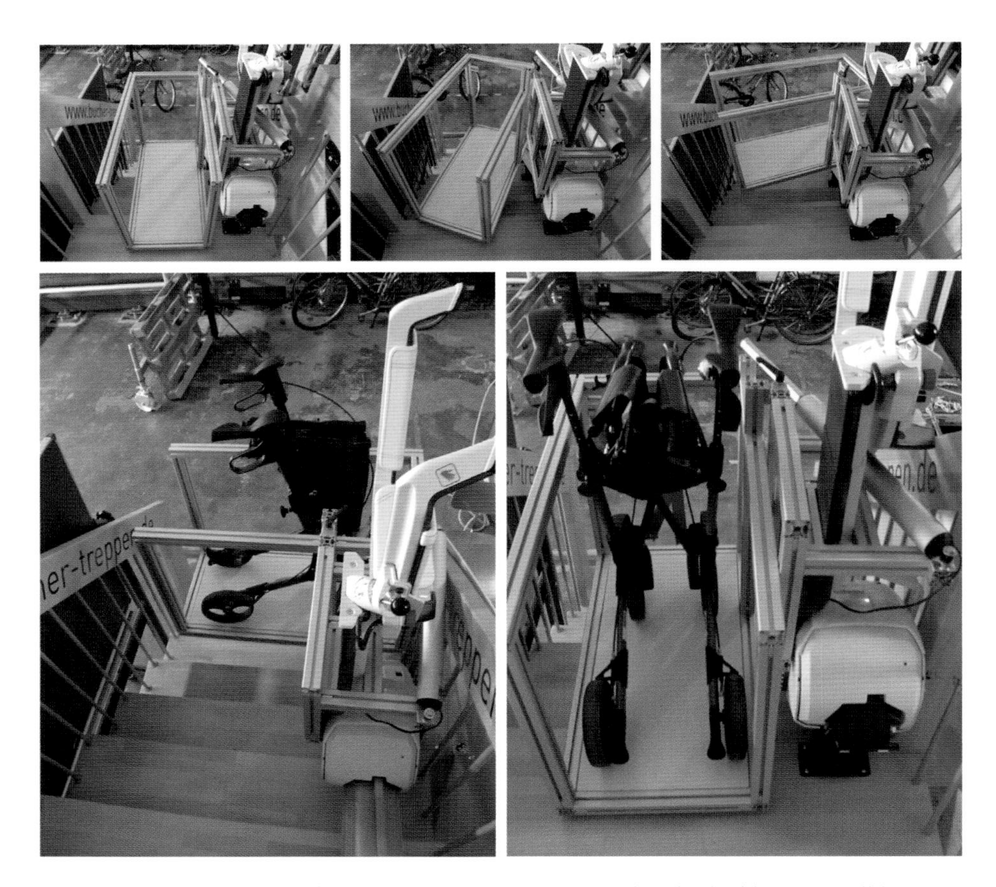

Figure 5.12 The StairWalker, including the transport box, synchronized with the overall home system, which allows the TurtleBot to remotely control the system.

own. The device just supports stair climbing, just like a rollator supports walking. Such devices are important to avoid an accelerated senescence, because if the elderly person continues to climb stairs, muscle will not begin to atrophy according to laws of nature – use it or lose it [163]. However, to enable the user (or the TurtleBot) to leave the apartment with the rollator, an automated transport box has been added, which is 100 percent with the overall indoor system.

This means that the GUI, and also the end user, is able to control the StairWalker and the TurtleBot. Depending on the source code, the TurtleBot is potentially able to call the appropriate shell script commands, depending on his current position on the apartment map. The details on how the interface between the tablet, or smartphone, and the robot has been realized is described by [164].

These prototypical implementations, which have been tested by the elderly in the laboratory test apartment, allowed to simulate several solutions as depicted in Figure 5.13.

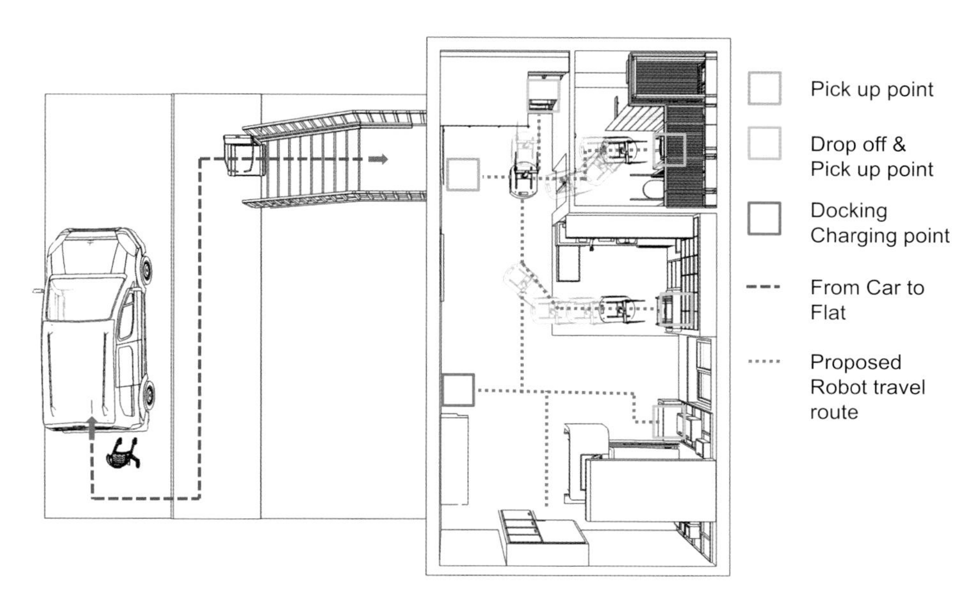

Figure 5.13 Simulation results of possibilities by the introduced technical solutions.

Using stronger robots than the TurtleBot would also add the simulated tasks. Depending on the robots' oriented design, the mobile platform, e.g., the Lynx Adept, could be enabled to carry objects to the car or into the apartment. For this purpose, special add-ons have been designed, as depicted in Figure 5.14.

5.4 Project USA²

Project USA² (**U**biquitäres und **S**elbstbestimmtes **A**rbeiten im **A**lter) aimed to develop decentralized work stations, which allow the retired elderly (or fragile) to take active part in the work life. The project focused on retired engineers for a period of one year with support of up to € 300,000 from the BMBF. Figure 5.15 demonstrates the basic idea of this project.

As it can be seen in Figure 5.15, this project considered the whole lifecycle of the product, starting with the product planning, development, quality security and testing up to service support. By recording and sharing the knowledge, robotic elements should learn basic movements or tasks, in order to support the elderly. The prototype concept was developed for three different scenarios: (a) for use as a modern production station in companies, (b) for home use, and (c) for use in "Brainspots." A Brainspot can be seen as a decentralized manufacturing corner, where the companies and communities provide the elderly in a neighborhood access to this workstation to allow them to stay active in their former employment.

At the same time in countries like Germany, it is expected that by 2030, approximately 7 million fewer employees will exist as compared to today. This means that

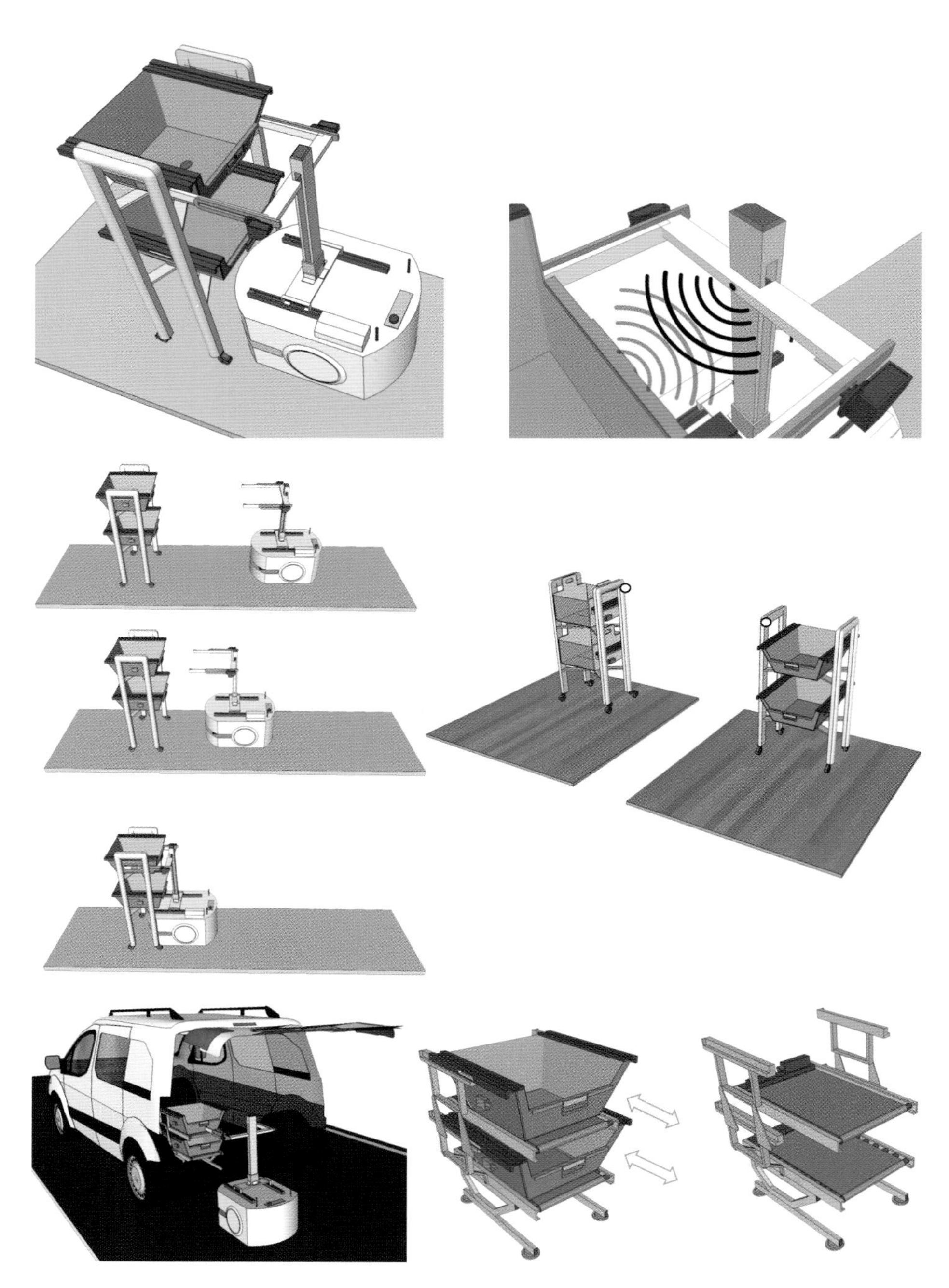

Figure 5.14 Apartment/car shelf storage systems, robot oriented designed in order to have a maximal compatibility regarding automated indoor/car storing.

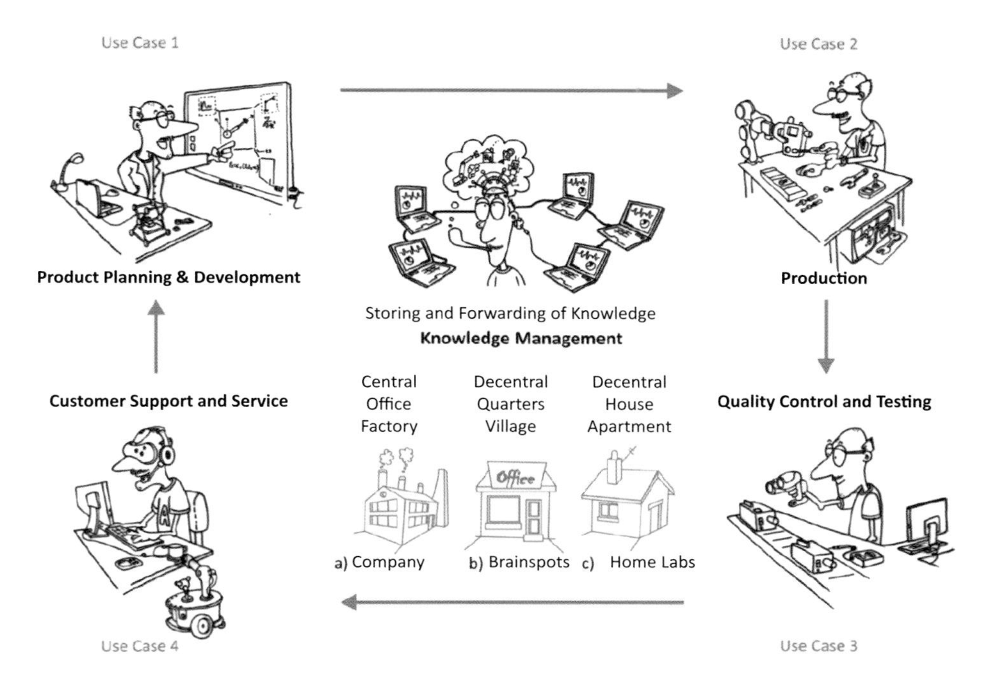

Figure 5.15 Structure representing the basic project idea using a scenario, and the product lifecycle model, which has been investigated by the prototype developed in the project.

within the next years, the gross national product will reduce by 16 percent [165], including a large knowledge loss, because of the retirement of highly experienced employees. There are existing studies (e.g., [166]), which prove the abilities of the "young." By keeping the elderly person especially mentally active, the process of senility should be slowed down [167], [168]. This means that this approach leads to a "win-win-situation", as the economy together with the elderly and their health benefit.

In order to allow for a proof of concept laboratory test, new technologies like 3D scanning and 3D printing, have been used for the production. Also, in this "mini home-factory," robots support the work. A robotic arm (Jaco-arm robot [169]) and a logistic platform (for this basic investigation the TurtleBot has been used) have been implemented in the work station.

The overall shape of the workstation orientates on the ergonomic structure of an airplane cockpit. The pilot in an airplane cockpit can easily reach each important switch. This leads to the specific design of the decentralized mini home-factory, as shown in Figure 5.16.

The basic frame has been designed using Maytec profiles. The surrounding shape, including the user head structure, allow the future inclusion of modules for different tasks. Furthermore, the workplace can be segmented in four different areas, where for each area, a different main task was conceived (as presented in Figure 5.17).

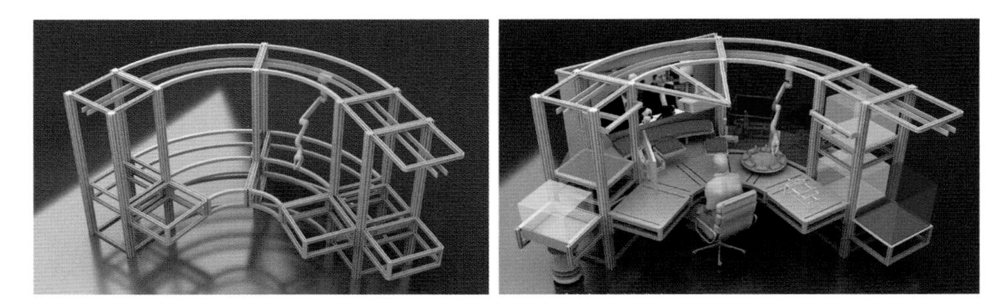

Figure 5.16 Design of the "mini home-factory." Left: the frame constructed by Maytec profiles. Right: the basic thoughts about modules (teleconference, robots, manufacturing, and 3D scanning tools) and their inclusion.

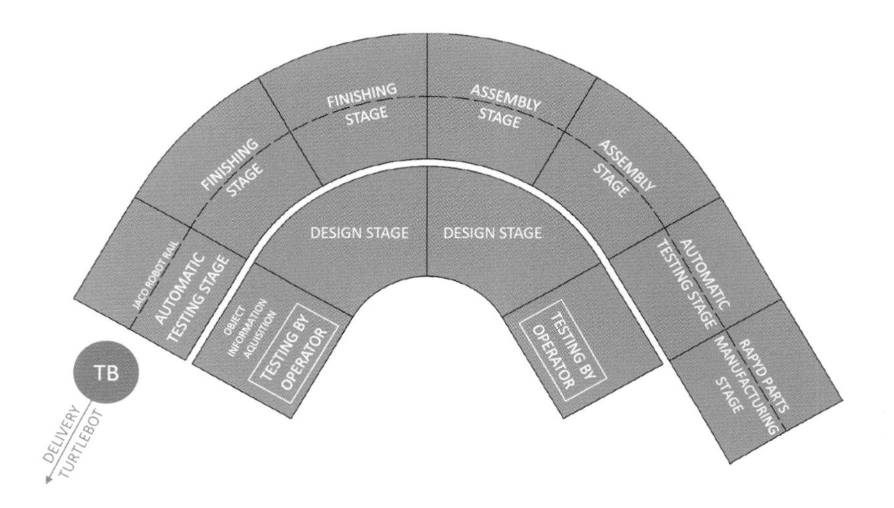

Figure 5.17 The different segments of the "mini home-factory," with their task objectives.

The front table also serves as a security obstacle, as it blocks the user from easily reaching the back area of the workstation where the automated testing, finishing, assembly, etc., takes place. The reason therefore is the idea that in this area where automated processes take place, the user can easily be harmed (e.g., by accidents or by misuse).

The prototype depicted in Figure 5.18 has been built in order to investigate the possible integration of different modules which will lead to the mini home-factory.

The workplace aimed to enable elderly engineers (from different fields) to stay active (or become active again) in society. Figure 5.19 shows how the workplace will be implemented, and represents the whole production cycle of a customized handgrip of a walking aid.

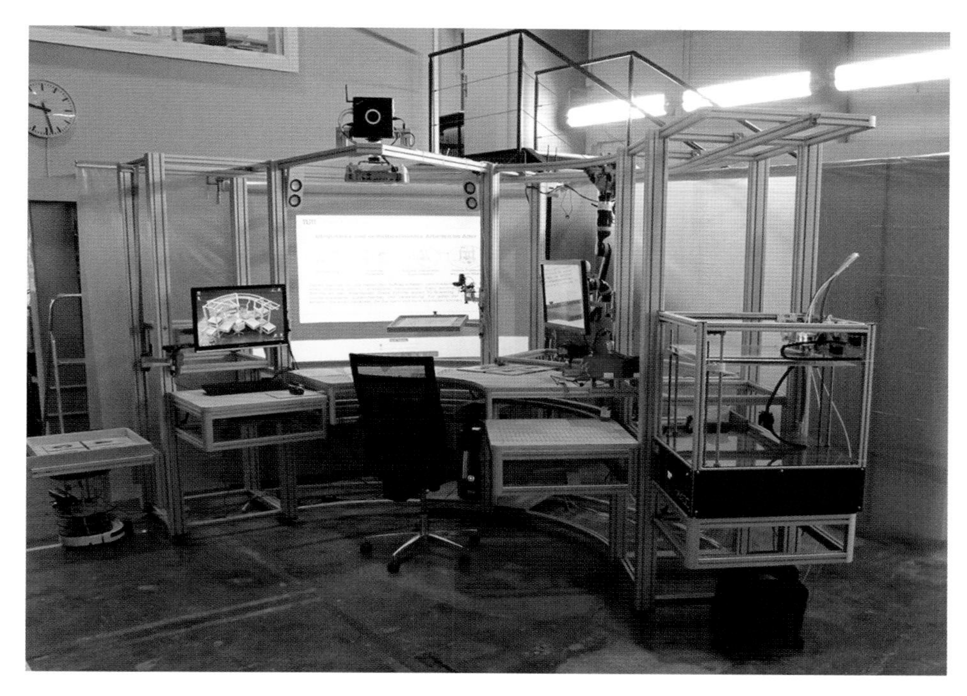

Figure 5.18 Developed "mini home-factory" of the project USA².

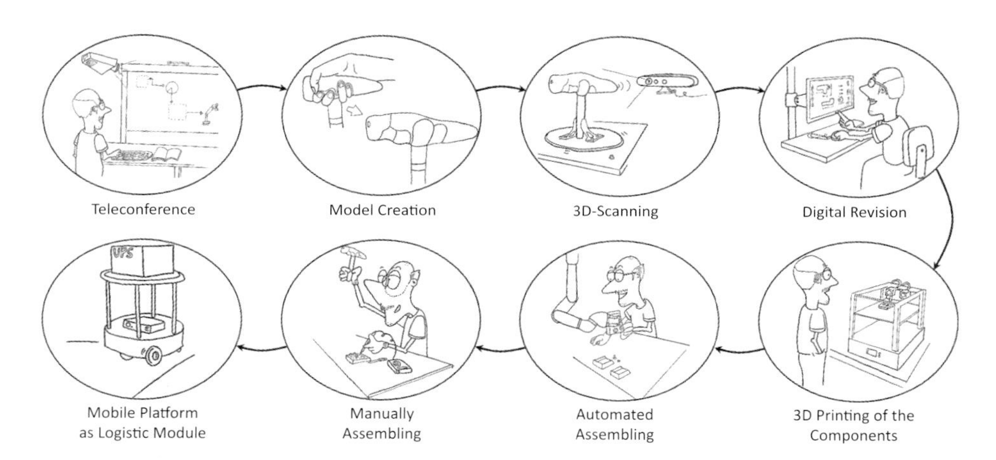

Figure 5.19 The production of an item using the mini home-factory; the process starts with the teleconference module (to receive instructions), followed by building an initial model that will be scanned using 3D scanning technology, and finally digital improvement and adjustment of the scanned result.

The user may attend work tasks, production discussions as well as meetings via the telepresence module consisting of a beamer, a beamer wall, and two HD webcams. The two cameras are necessary because of the possibility to sketch something (e.g., on a sheet of paper) and to immediately show it on a specific table to the audience by using

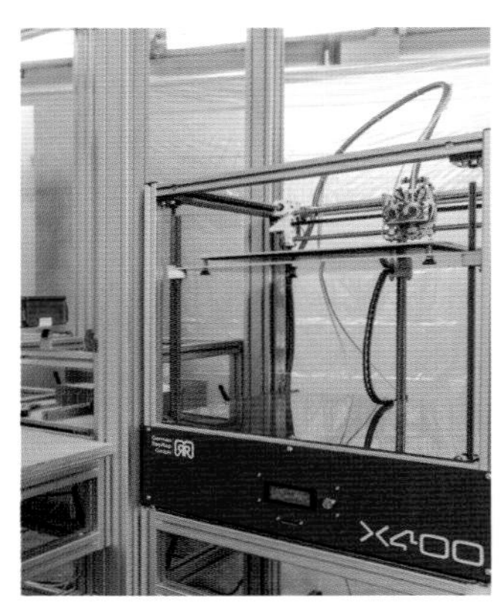

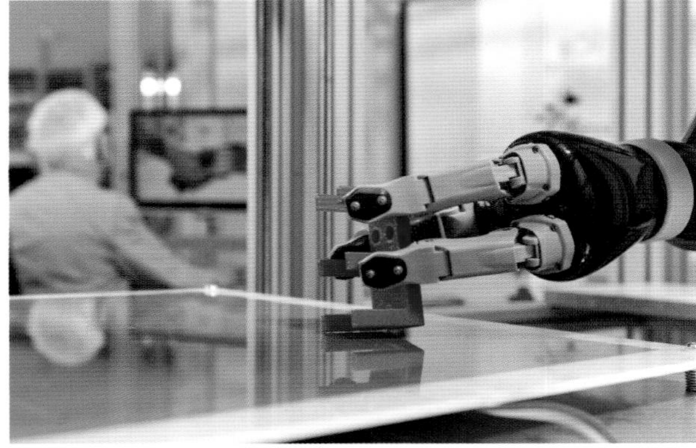

Figure 5.20 Left: 3D Printer X400 from German RepRap. Right: the 3D Pinter interacting with the robotic arm Jaco.

picture-in-picture mode. As soon as the user knows the work task, the preparation of a model using CAD software is necessary. In order to allow an easy and fast modeling process, e.g., by using a small scaled sample, the user could scan the object and immediately receive the basic contour data.

For the manufacturing, a 3D printer (German RepRap X400) has been used. A robotic arm on the rail could drive to the printer and grasp in it, in order to transport the object to the user (as depicted in Figure 5.20). To manage the transport of materials or the final product, a logistic platform was used.

In order to allow the user to interact with this backstage area without coming too close to it, the robotic arm, Jaco, services as a secure interface. Jaco is mounted (as depicted in Figures 5.16 and 5.18) on a rail at the top of the workstation. From here, the arm can move in each of the back segments of the "mini home-factory."

Even today where the use of technology and robotics is much easier than 40 years ago, it can be challenging for an elderly person to efficiently use a robotic arm. An intuitive control option had to be found. Three different control options (automated tasks, virtual joystick, and gesture control) for the robotic arm have been implemented and their user acceptance further investigated in a laboratory test. The overall control, where the user decides the most preferred control, is depicted in Figure 5.21.

The control option to use automated task and the joystick control represents already known control options. The gesture control represents a new innovative way to control the robotic arm (visible in Figure 5.22). The Leap motion sensor has been used as an interface to recognize the user hand and send the movement information to the robotic arm [169]. This allows an intuitive use of the robot, which elderly of all education classes can use.

Nevertheless, the complexity of the possibilities of this workplace was still so large (comparable with the complexity of a car) that the user requires guidelines. Therefore, the Augmented Reality Device, Vuzix, has been used (visible in Figure 5.23). By contour recognition, as well as 2D barcodes, the Vuzix M100 could instruct the user on how to use the different applications (e.g., by tutorials with the loudspeaker and the display), giving hints as to where the switches are, etc. [170].

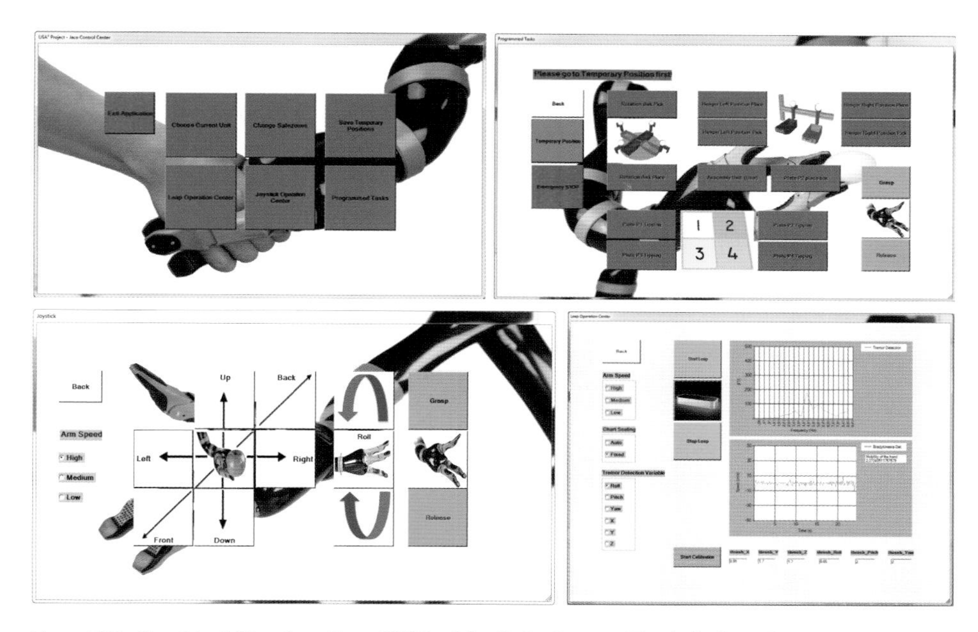

Figure 5.21 Graphical User Interface (GUI) of the Robotic arm. Top left: Start GUI, where the user selects the control mechanism, Top right: GUI allows execution of automated tasks, Bottom left: GUI allows to directly navigate the robot by arrow buttons, Bottom right: GUI allows arm control by gesture, the GUI displays the physiological measurements which are executed in parallel.

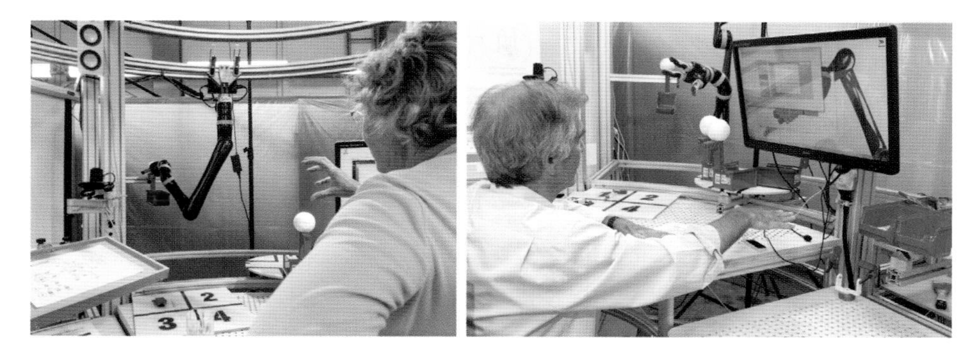

Figure 5.22 Gesture control of the robotic arm Jaco.

This system offered a unique opportunity to implement a physiological measurement. While the user is working with the robots using gestures (this keeps the elderly active and healthy) and gets guidelines by the AR device Vuzix M100, the tremor of the head and the hand can be analyzed [170], [171]. This is possible as the Vuzix M100 has gyroscopes and accelerometers implemented. For hand analysis, a numerical differentiation is necessary to receive the user hand movement acceleration from the position values of the hand. The measurement possibility has been demonstrated by display of the appropriated GUI as shown in Figure 5.24.

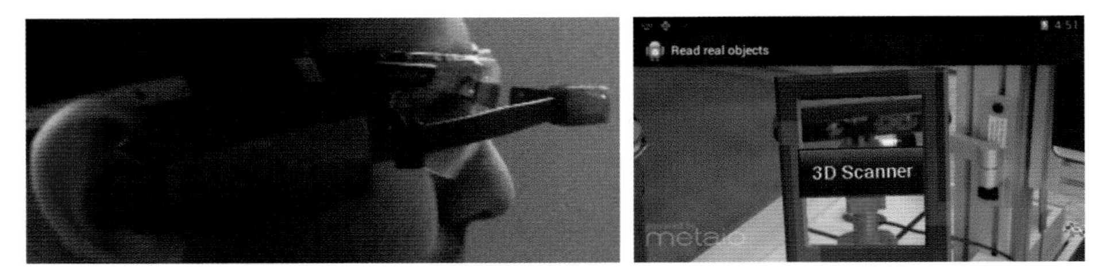

Figure 5.23 Left: Vuzix M100. Right: The augmented reality information about the 3D scanner camera.

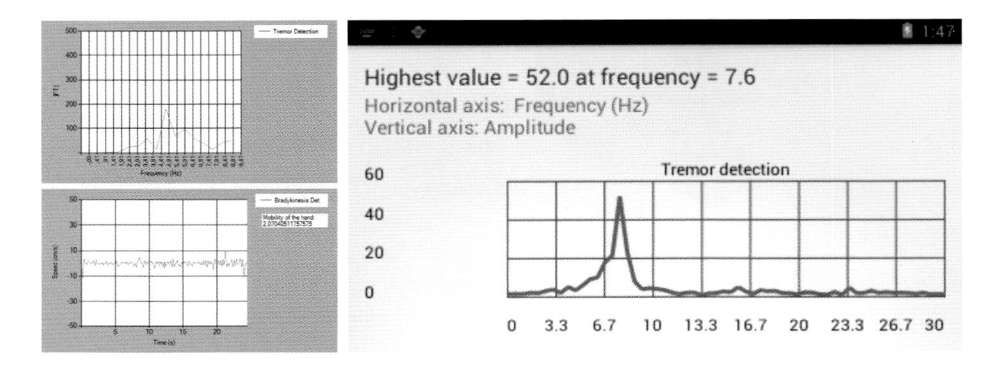

Figure 5.24 Visual result of the tremor analysis and the bradykinesia detection of the Leap Motion sensor (left), and on the right, the head tremor analysis by the Vuzix M100.

On a second stage, in order to estimate a possible bradykinesia, not only the tremor, but also the speed of movement was analyzed according to A. Salarian et al. [172].

The information about tremor and bradykinesia of elderly is of interest because they are indicators of nerve diseases like Parkinson's disease [173]. These diseases mainly affect elderly above 55 years (i.e., the target user group) and the prevalence has increased over the last years.

Furthermore, Parkinson's is not the only disease that can cause symptoms like tremors. Several diseases may also lead to these symptoms, but they differ in their frequencies and amplitudes, e.g., essential tremors [173]. By recording the analysis of the user movements and combining with telemedical applications, an early intervention can be realized in the future. This would increase the life quality mainly because currently there is no known recovery method for diseases such as Parkinson's, as it is only possible to slow down their progress. Therefore, the earliest the intervention process starts, the more that life quality in old age can be secured.

5.5 Project LISA-Habitec

The project LISA-habitec (Living independently in Südtirol Alto-Adige through an Integration of Habitat, Assistance, Bits and Technology by a value System based on

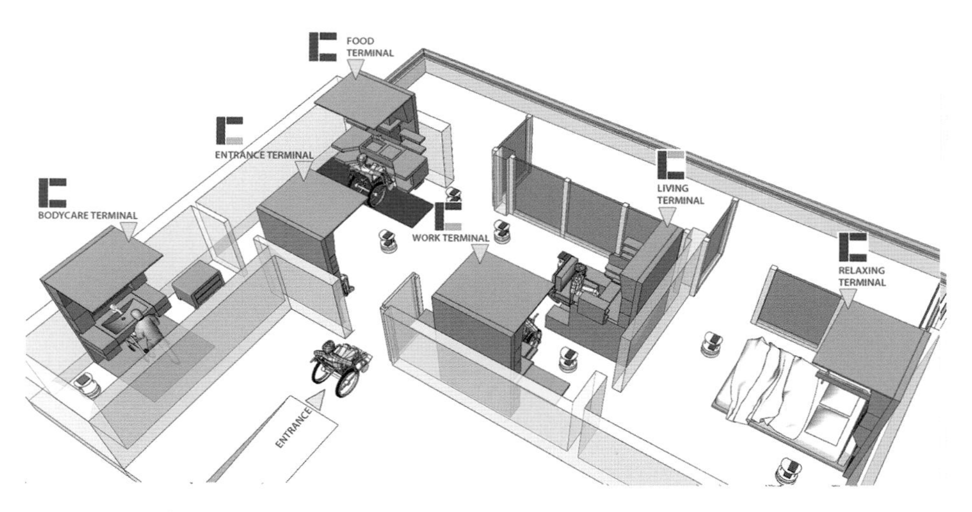

Figure 5.25 Basic concept of the LISA-habitec smart AAL walls.

local Resources) is a follow-up project based on LISA (see Section 5.2). In this project, not only one apartment area is considered (as in LISA), but rather a smart LISA AAL wall for all apartment areas is developed. The predefined apartment areas from LISA have been incorporated into this project, including the knowledge about the necessary space which enabled understanding of the basic concepts at the start of the project (Figure 5.25).

Here, the most challenging aspect for each apartment is to define the area specific service function which allows the elderly to even stay alone at home. For this purpose, a basic analysis was done at the very beginning of the project. The elderly both at home and in care homes were asked about their preferred support and needs.

Table 5.1 gives an overview about the potential functions and service modules considered from the beginning. Additionally, user benefit has been evaluated by interviewing the elderly.

Once all potential service functions were collected, they were additionally analyzed according to innovation, technical feasibility, expected material, and production costs, expected benefits to all stakeholders etc. This approach allowed for ranking of the collected ideas regarding the service modules. The objective in the project was to come up with three new and highly innovative functions for each apartment area. The smart LISA AAL walls would offer new functions without staying in competition with already existing products.

Within this project, several prototypes as shown in Figure 5.26 have been developed.

The kitchen and bathroom areas showed that it is more useful to develop a table and bed containing the different modular service functions instead of developing a smart AAL LISA wall.

Additionally, to this overall shape development, several service modules were also developed. These included new service module prototypes that give the smart environment an advantage over its competitors. These newly invented prototypical service modules are describedin the next section.

Table 5.1 Service Functions of the Different Smart AAL LISA Walls – Bathroom and Kitchen

	Service Functions	User Benefit
Basic Wall	Emergency call	5
	Fall detection	5
	Medication dispenser	3
	Vital data measurement	3
	Communication	4
	User interface	4
	Central controlling unit/house technic	3
	Data platform for access of several user	4
	Multifunctional robot	3
Bath room	Sink	3
	Mirror	3
	Storage options/bathroom cabinet	3
	Towel rail	3
	Handles and rods to hold on	4
	Height adjustability	4
	Light and lightning atmosphere	3
	Module for cleaning denture, teeth brush, etc.	3
	Assistance with reaching objects	3
	Heat radiation	4
	Seating accommodation	4
	Module for measuring weight/body fat, BMI, temperature	3
	Overflow sensor	4
	Automated regulation of the sink water temperature	4
	Automated regulation of the water temperature	4
	Support with applying cream	4
	Full body dryer	4
Kitchen	Automated shut down of devices	5
	Automated detection of security relevant environmental parameters	5
	Seating accommodation	4
	Height adjustability	4
	Repair and maintenance services	3
	Integration of eating opportunity	3
	Assistance in serving food	3
	Light and lightning atmosphere	3
	Dispenser/magazine for liquids	3
	Cooking machine	3
	Module for the automated cutting of food	3
	Automated reordering of food/catering services	2
	Assistance with reaching objects	3

5.5.1 Coat Dressing Aid

In old age, wearing the correct cloth is quite important. For example, wearing a very thin coat in winter can trigger influenza, which is faster and easily distributed nowadays. For the elderly, this is very risky [174]. Often, some have to briefly leave the apartment (e.g., to throw away garbage). If it is too exhausting, painful, or difficult to slip into a

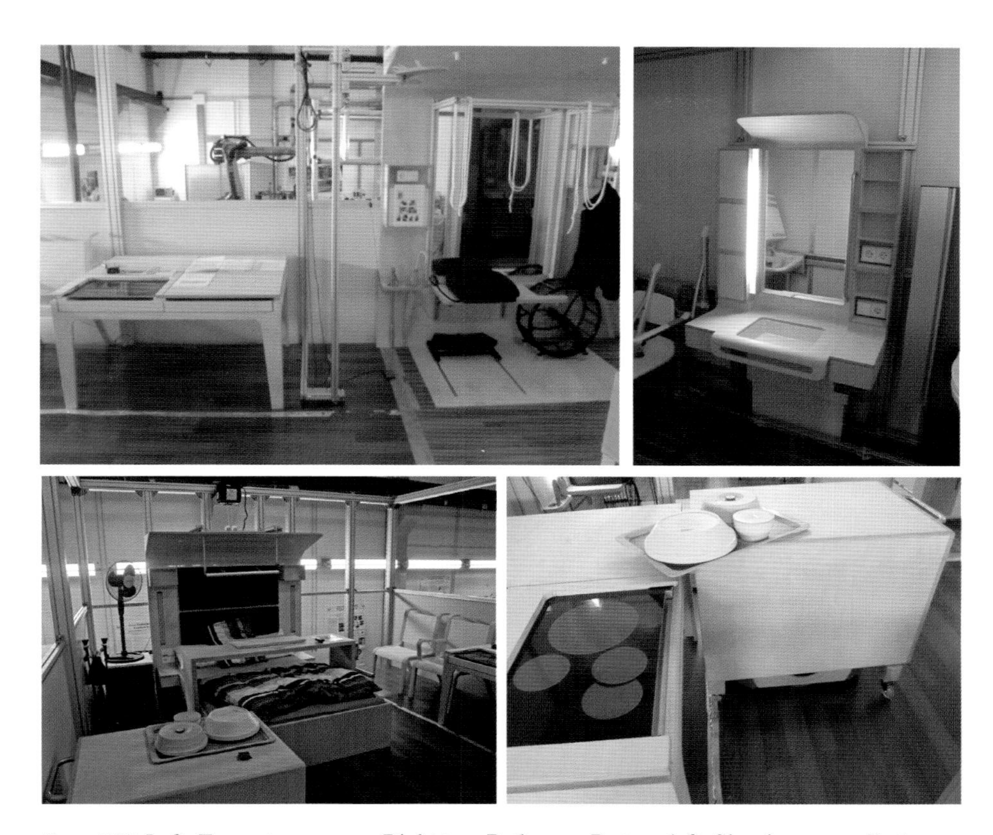

Figure 5.26 Left: Top entrance area. Right top: Bath area. Bottom left: Sleeping room. Bottom right: Kitchen.

coat, the elderly will go out without one. The cold makes people rush and in worst cases may lead to accidents. Once the mobility decreases, as expected while aging, wearing a coat becomes challenging. Age-related diseases like Parkinson's and osteoporosis can lead to the necessity of requiring a second person (helper/care giver) to dress the affected elderly when the need arises. Also, in old age, the elderly will sooner or later be alone, and this aspect can already lead to a dependency that can only be properly treated in a care home. Therefore, the prototype shown in Figure 5.27 has been developed.

With this device, only minor dexterity is needed to put on the coat. A foot switch triggers the device, which then drives to the user in order to attach the coat. As soon as this is done, the senior lays his or her hands in the coat arms and presses the foot switch again. By appropriate driving of the two actuators attached at the top, the coat gets drawn up and moves forward at the end, and the user attaches the coat using the clamps. Therefore, the coat first gets laid on the device as shown in Figure 5.27. This allows the device to clamp the collar using clips. Once this is done, the coat will hang on the device and follow the body contour. The device must be setup individually to the user's height. At the end of the procedure, the

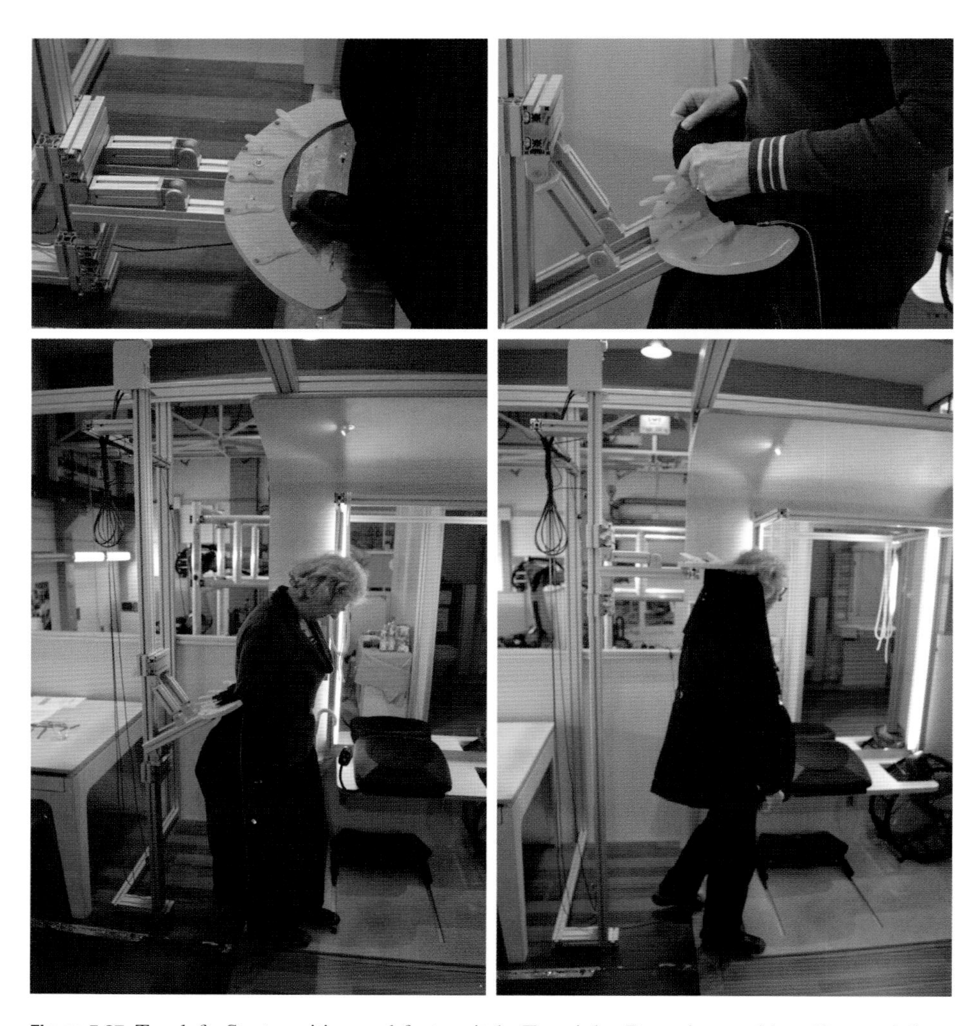

Figure 5.27 Top left: Start position and foot switch. Top right: Preparing position. Bottom left: Starting the dress support mechanism. Bottom right: Automated dress support completed.

user presses the foot switch in order to move the device to its parking position at the very top. By applying force on the clips, the collar slips out and the user can continue with his business.

5.5.2 Contactless Fever Measuring

Health is of major importance to those who are fragile, and it is therefore advantageous to know about their current health conditions. For example, fever mostly occurs when the immune system is defending the body against pathogens [175]. Recording body temperature over time gives a summary of health condition developments and aids in the prevention of complications, e.g., to avoid developing pneumonia following a minor

Max. Temp.: 36.5 ¦ Min. Temp.: 26.3
Temperatur: 36.38 Pixelwert: 252 Koordinaten: [31, 61]
Max. Temp.: 36.7 ¦ Min. Temp.: 26.4
Temperatur: 36.4576 Pixelwert: 249 Koordinaten: [32, 63]
Max. Temp.: 36.6 ¦ Min. Temp.: 26.3
Temperatur: 36.398 Pixelwert: 250 Koordinaten: [31, 62]
Max. Temp.: 36.6 ¦ Min. Temp.: 26.3
Temperatur: 36.398 Pixelwert: 250 Koordinaten: [31, 62]
Max. Temp.: 36.5 ¦ Min. Temp.: 26.2
Temperatur: 36.3384 Pixelwert: 251 Koordinaten: [31, 61]
Max. Temp.: 36.5 ¦ Min. Temp.: 26.2
Temperatur: 36.298 Pixelwert: 250 Koordinaten: [30, 60]
Max. Temp.: 36.5 ¦ Min. Temp.: 26.1
Temperatur: 36.1329 Pixelwert: 246 Koordinaten: [33, 65]
Max. Temp.: 36.5 ¦ Min. Temp.: 26.2
Temperatur: 35.8537 Pixelwert: 239 Koordinaten: [33, 65]
Temperatur Mittelwert: 36.0193
Standardabweichung: 0.552338
Koerpertemperatur: 36.1814

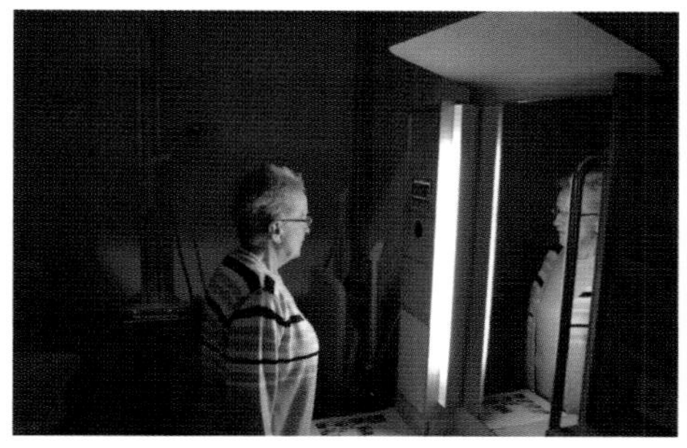

Figure 5.28 Left: The unobtrusive measurement of body temperature. Right: Display of the results for demonstration purposes.

infection. Although everyone in their life has had their body temperature measured, there is a possibility of making mistakes in the measurement. Furthermore, measuring fever can be time consuming, making it very inconvenient to track body temperature. Meanwhile, there exists several devices which can measure body temperature on the forehead or ear drum via infrared [176], [177], [178]. Nevertheless, who has time and the intention to track the measurements frequently over days and weeks? Additionally, hygiene must be considered, especially when the device is used on several people [179].

Therefore, a module for contactless fever measurement has been developed. As shown in Figure 5.28, this module is hidden inside the smart LISA AAL bath wall.

The module permanently tries to measure body temperature; as soon as a human face is detected, the device searches for the forehead and captures the temperature. To do this, a thermal camera is used. For the forehead finding algorithm, a single-board computer (BeagleBone Black) has been connected to the thermal camera to read out the images and carry out analysis (see Figure 5.29).

In order to avoid many wrong measurements, several measurements are detected and analyzed but get cancelled for the final result calculation according to stray bullet (see Figure 5.28). The display serves just for demonstration (or prototypical) purposes. In order to enable the module, the modular interface ability, as in Section 5.1, an XBee antenna has been attached.

XBee antennas, when compared to Bluetooth and Wi-Fi, operate on the principles of radio waves, and have a much larger transmission distance. Like Wi-Fi and Bluetooth, this module offers access securities like ID numbers, passwords, and encryption of the transmitted data. Their high transmission distance and small size allows a straight forward, and according to their lower popularity compared to Wi-Fi, more secure wireless data transmission.

Details regarding the development and the functionality of the contactless fever measurement for this specific purpose can be read in [180].

5.5.3 Contactless ECG Measuring

The possibility to measure unobtrusively and without any direct contact has many advantages. However, this is not possible in most cases. For example, in ECG

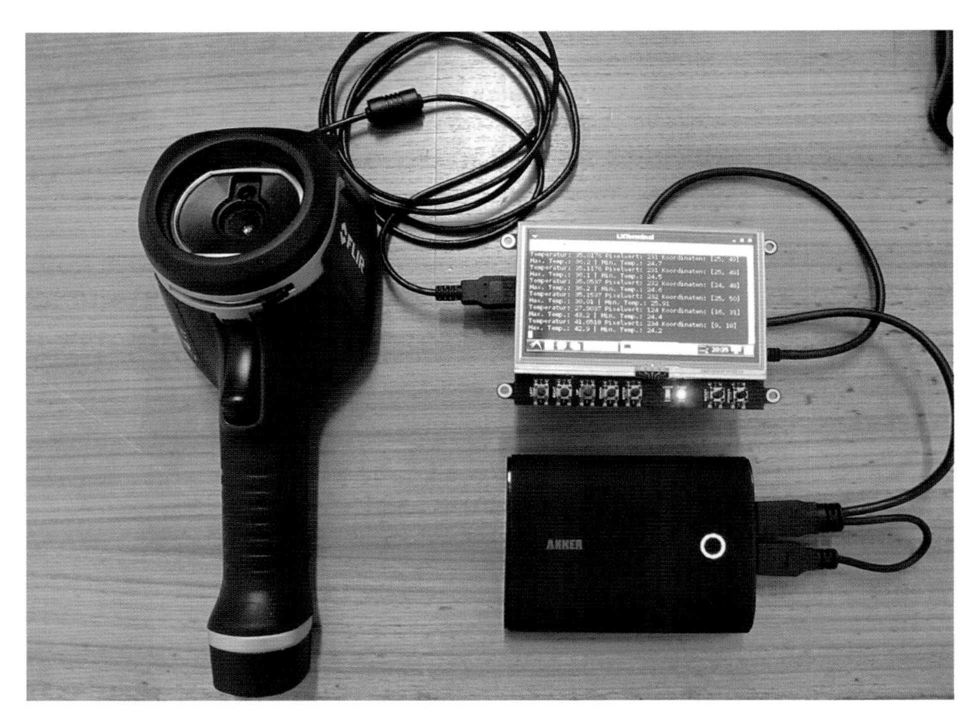

Figure 5.29 The fever measurement system, powered by a battery.

measurements, which belongs to one of the most common and important measurements in medicine, there does not exists a way to measure without contact. Normally, at least three to four electrodes (for one to six leads, see Chapter 2) which must be placed at appropriate spots in order to enable a comparable measurement are necessary.

Skin irritations are often the result of the self-holding glue electrodes. Therefore, capacitive electrodes are of high interest for the project. They have the potential to measure the ECG even through clothes. To verify this, a prototype using the Beagle-Bone Black for the user interface, Arduino with appropriate ECG shield (ECG shield from Olimex), and capacitive electrodes has been used to investigate the use of this technology in the home environment (see Figure 5.30).

As soon as the prototype was set up, it was implemented in a wooden armchair as shown in Figure 5.31.

For this system, two electrode chips (PS25203B and PS25201B) were purchased and compared. The instigation of their potential regarding ECG signal quality (depicted in Figure 5.32) shows that at direct skin contact, the signal quality is even much better than using normal electrodes. Additionally, measuring through clothes is possible. Nevertheless, the electrodes are very sensitive and capture early noise (e.g., from the power sockets in the room). To avoid this issue, it is necessary to shield the system properly [181].

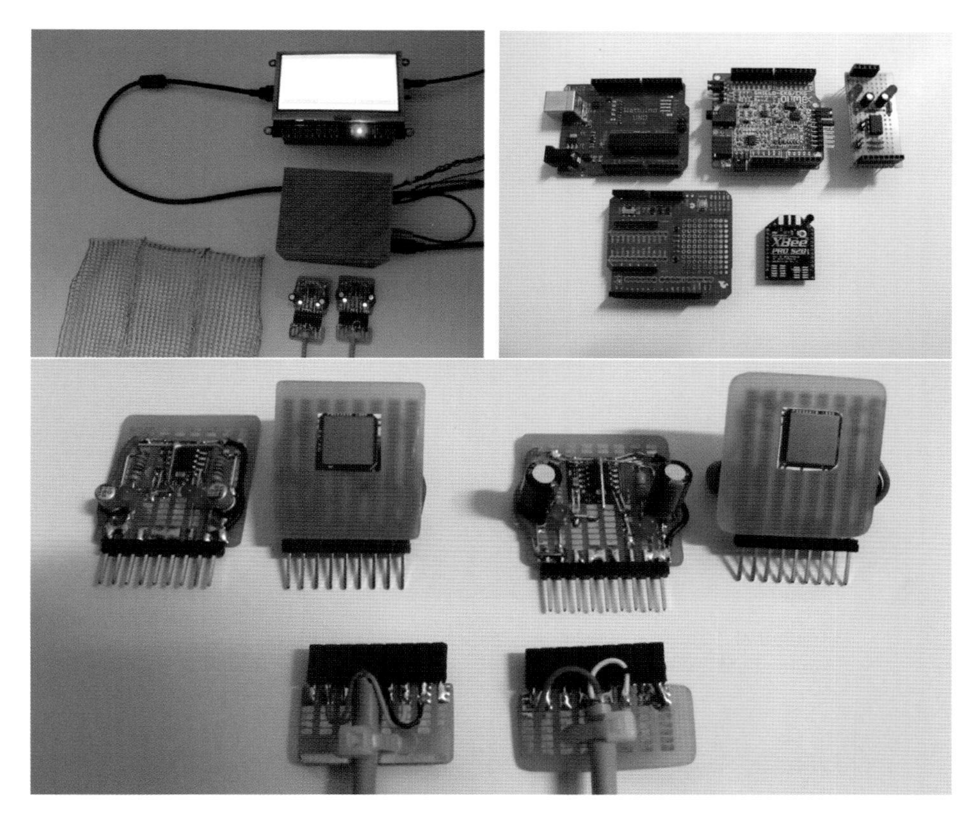

Figure 5.30 Top left: The capacitive ECG prototype. Top right: Wattuino, ECG shield and XBee shield, as well as drive ground plane circuit. Bottom: Capacitive electrodes as equalized interface to the prototype.

Here also, the XBee antennas were used in order to investigate the potential possibility for real-time data transmission. To do so, the ECG measurement was recorded and compared with different modular settings.

While the results showed that the XBee modules are able to measure, the data transmission is too slow and down samples the sample frequency. This sample frequency down sampling leads to a reduction in the signal resolution. The outcome is, as shown in Figure 5.33, that not all heart peaks can be reliably be detected. Therefore, instead of transmitting the whole ECG signal in real time, the XBee will focus on transmitting just the end results (e.g., the pulse). The BeagleBone Black is fortunately able to store the ECG signal, in order to allow a detail investigation if necessary. For this purpose, the stored data must be read out using, e.g., USB sticks.

5.5.4 Fall Detection

Falling is a major problem, even for the young and healthy. However, falling risk increases in old age due to balance issues. Several systems to detect a fall exist (e.g.,

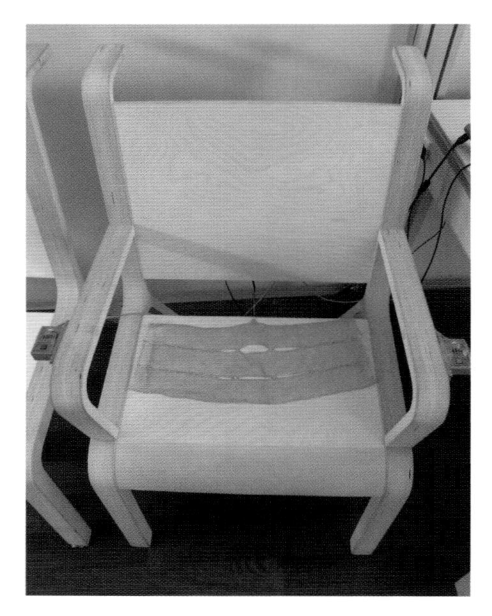

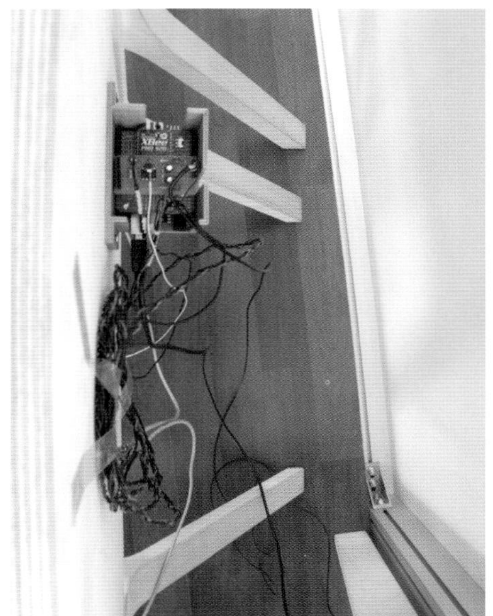

Figure 5.31 Left: front side of the implemented capacitive ECG. Right: the unobtrusive attachment on the back of the chair.

accelerometers and gyroscopes). Such systems can be implemented in mobile phones and smartphones as well as in augmented reality devices (e.g., VUZIX M100). Also, sensor mates and "SensFloor" exist [182]. However, SensFloor is the only system which is not a wearable but can reliably detect a fall. Wearables and mates always have the risk that a person is either not wearing the device or is falling next to it.

The SensFloor is based on capacity, similar to smartphones. Unlike pressure sensors, the capacitive sensor is covered by the ground, which protects the sensible sensors. However, there is one big disadvantage: the SensFloor is not usable in the bath. Here, special water mates are necessary, but both approaches are costly, and therefore, a cost-efficient alternative has been investigated. The idea here was to use line lasers that can shoot on up to 15 photo resistors. These settings have been tested in a laboratory test apartment as depicted in Figure 5.34.

The photo resistors are attached to an ArduinoMega, which is directly connected to an XBee module that forward the information about a fall/not a fall to a server. For the prototype, red lasers were used in order to demonstrate the function (see Figure 5.34). However, in a real home environment, infrared lasers will be used.

In order to reduce the power consumption of the lasers, a transistor driven by the ArduinoMega control allows to switch the laser on, only for the measurement of how many resistors are blocked. If a specific amount is blocked, the system recognizes it as a fall, as it knows that only the blocking size of a human laying on the ground can be able to block these number of sensors. As shown in Figure 5.35, the overall system can easily be installed as a hidden entity.

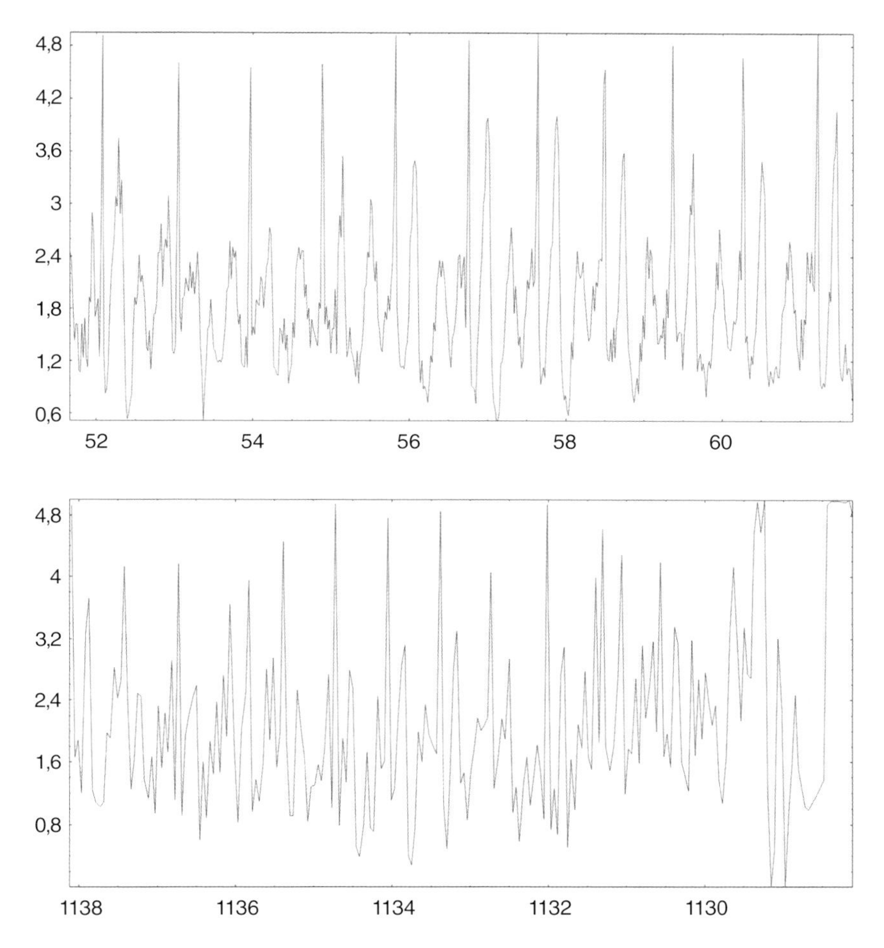

Figure 5.32 Top: ECG measurement with direct skin contact. Bottom: Measurement through a pullover on the chest.

5.5.5 Shoe Dressing Aid

Although the entrance area is already well covered with potential service modules (see Section 5.2), a special investigation has been done in the entrance area. The objective was to improve the shoe horn. For this purpose, a new kind of shoe shelf has been used. Under the seat of the elderly, a slide was developed which can drive up and enable the user to either put on or remove their shoes (see Figure 5.36).

The rotatory shoe shelf reduces the necessary space and allows an ergonomically easy way of reaching different types of shoes. Additionally, the seat offers support when standing up by use of a switch to the right of the user.

In the project, the potential use of an automated rotatory shelf and slide in combination with a belt lift system is investigated. This will not only allow to securely lift an

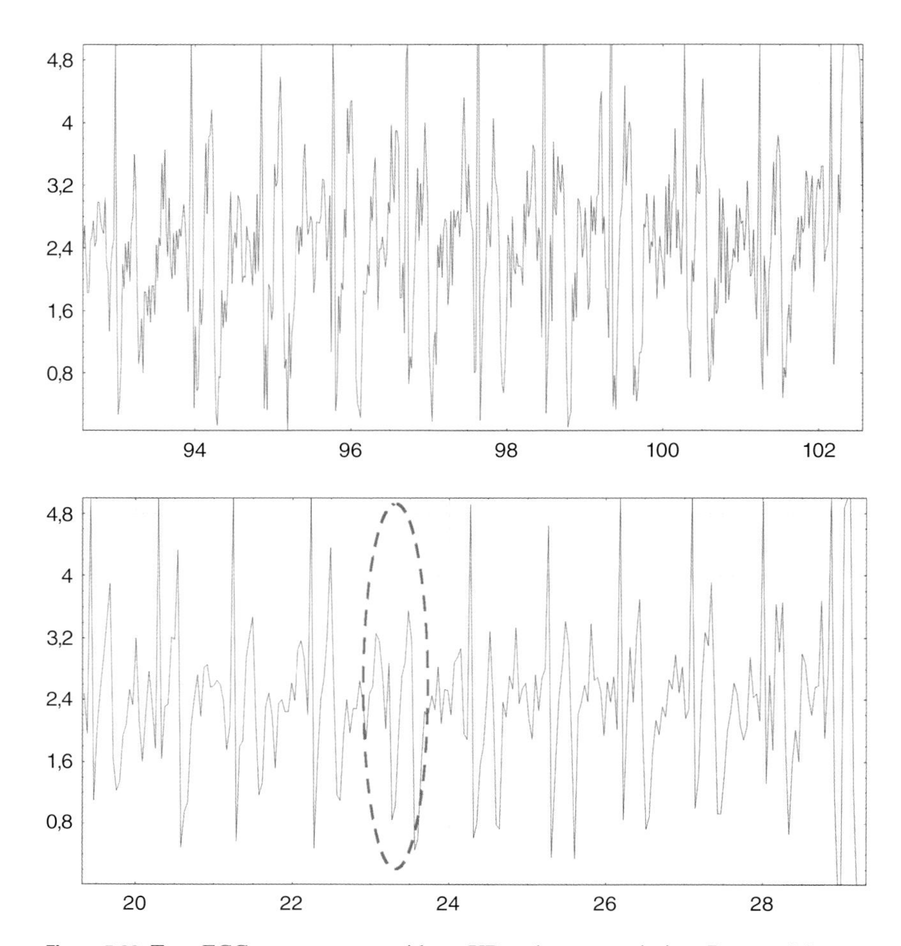

Figure 5.33 Top: ECG measurement without XBee data transmission. Bottom: Measurement with XBee data transmission.

elderly person but also to fully allow an automated shoe preparation step. As a result, this will support the elderly not only in the attract process but also in the shoe exhaust process as done in LISA (see Section 5.2).

5.5.6 Robotic Implementation

In the bedroom module, a drivable table which is thought to serve the user with space for books and tablets or laptops has been implemented. An included power supply socket allows laptops as well as table lamps to work directly in the bed. By automation, the user can drive the table in the appropriate position whenever he wants. As this table is fixed to the bed, only one-directional movements are possible. To automate this kind

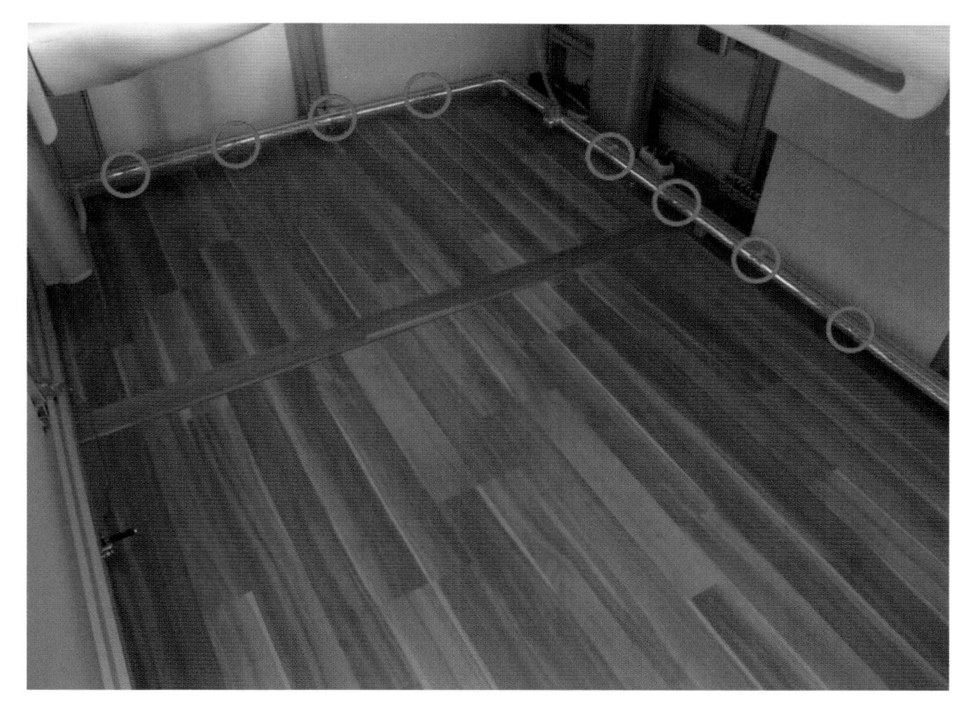

Figure 5.34 Photo resistors of the falling detection service module.

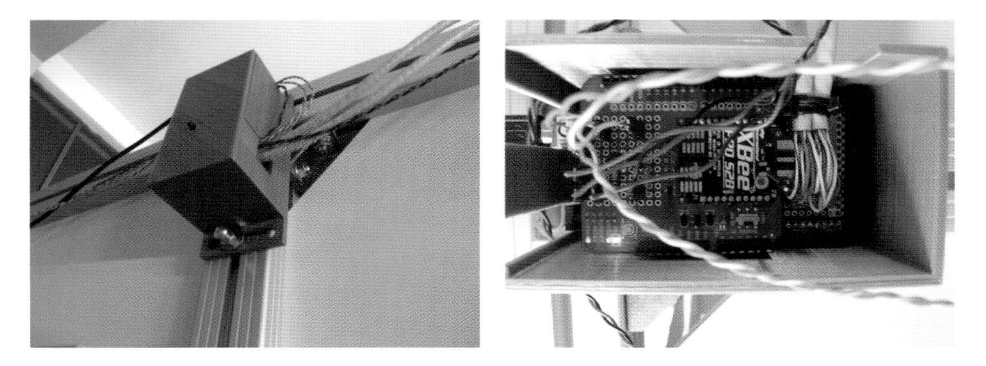

Figure 5.35 Left: The controlling unit unobtrusively attached on a wall. Right: In view of the controlling unit consisting of ArduinoMega, a shield for interfacing, and an XBee module.

of furniture is, therefore, compared to a kitchen table, easy. In Figure 5.37, a servant table is shown, which is thought to act as a mobile platform.

Since this set up means that both a two-dimensional movement and a larger payload is necessary, a strong mobile logistic robot is therefore needed. For this purpose, the PIONEER LX from adept mobile robots has been used. The robot is able to carry

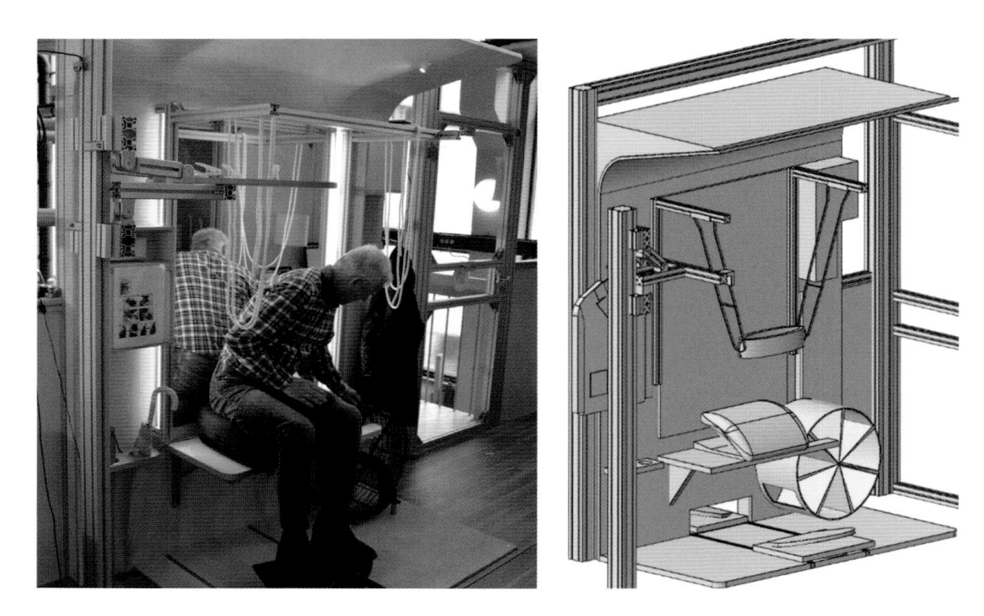

Figure 5.36 Left: Extended shoe support. Right: Overall concept including uplift belt.

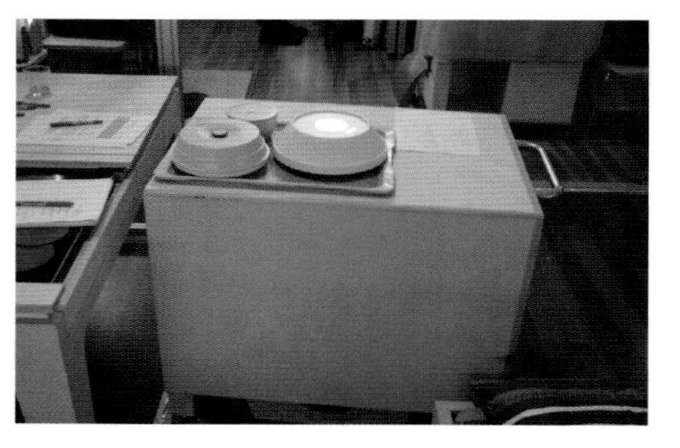

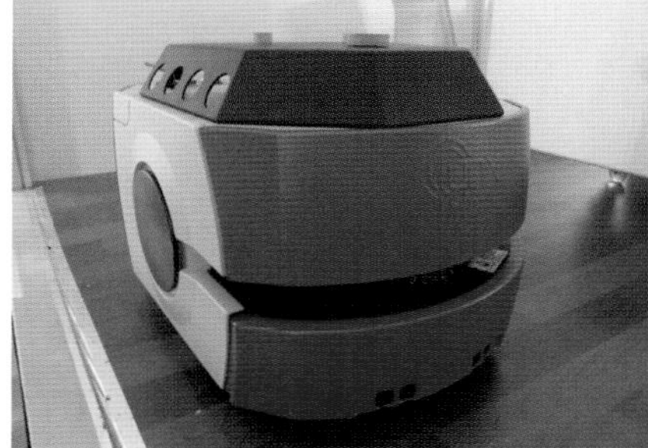

Figure 5.37 An automatic moving kitchen table (left) controlled by the robot shown on the right.

60 kg of payload, use a laser as well as four ultrasound sensors (onetime in front and onetime in the back) to avoid obstacles. To prevent the robot from crashing, a bumper in the front immediately stops the current movement. Unfortunately, the introducing interviews (regarding the potential service functions, summarized in Table 5.1) led to the finding that the elderly do not like robots, which obviously seem to be a complex technology (Table 5.2).

It can be assumed that in the next 20–50 years, the attitudes about robots may change. Currently, one solution to this issue is to integrate the robot into a table. As a result, the concerns over robots in the home decreased (the result of a laboratory test),

Table 5.2 Service Functions of the Different Smart AAL LISA Walls – Bed Room and Entrance Area

	Service functions	User benefit
Bed room	Interactive cooking/working surface	2
	Dressing support	4
	Wall-ceiling-element	4
	Bed	4
	Air purifier, temperature regulation	3
	Standing up/transfer support	3
	Support with daily preparing/cleaning of the bed	3
	To the annual season adaptable light	3
	Apartment access control	3
	Fall asleep support (by music etc.)	3
	Awakening support (e.g., wake up light)	3
	Design advisor	2
	Measurement of sleeping silence relevant data	2
Entrance area	Putting shoes on support	4
	Function for putt on clothes	4
	Remembering while forgetting important objects	3
	Ceiling or wall element with mirror	3
	Navigation support	3
	Seat accommodation	3
	Stand-assist	3
	Opening and closing door support	3
	Support in receiving of goods	3
	Remembering or automated shut down of devices	5

and the mobile table could function in the home in the same way. However, when integrating furniture, it is necessary that needed security sensors (i.e. bumper, ultrasound, and laser) are not covered.

To enable intuitive control of the robot by the elderly, a very simple GUI with large buttons has been realized and finally implemented in the BealgeBone Black (see Figure 5.38).

The weak point of this GUI in a real implementation is that the user needs more options in order to navigate the robot; this will in turn reduce the button size (until a larger screen is attached).

5.6 Project REACH

REACH (Responsive Engagement of the Elderly Promoting Activity and Customized Healthcare) is a project for personalized prevention and intervention systems that aim increasing quality of live in old age. For this purpose, sensor networks will be implemented in a user-friendly manner in the environment of the end user to analyze their habits and health condition. The combination of unobtrusive implemented sensors in the environment, wearables, and the actively measured results (blood pressure meter, etc.),

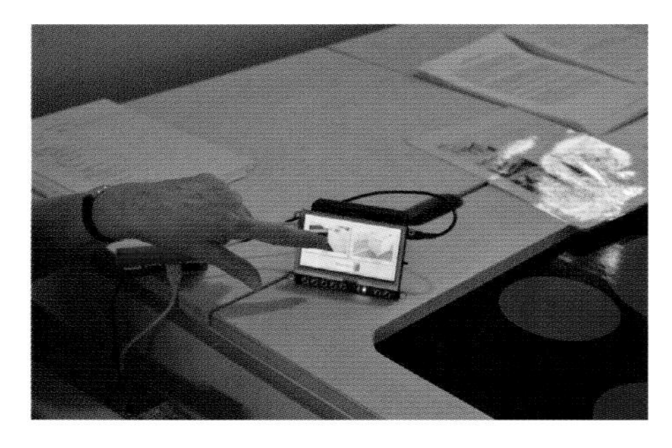

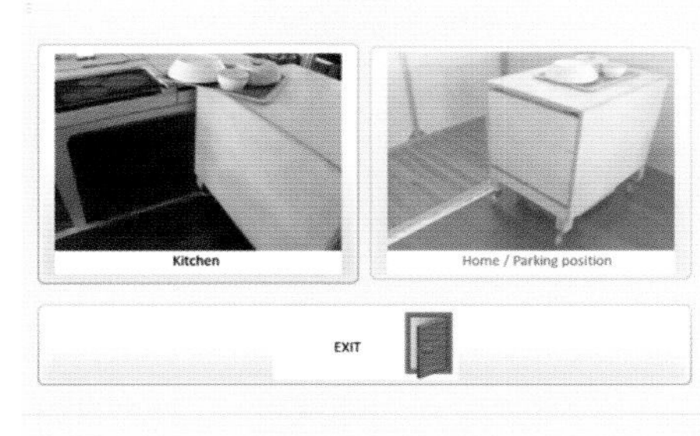

Figure 5.38 The BeagleBone Black (left) while an elderly person is using the GUI (depicted on the right) to control the kitchen table.

allow a seamless flow of information which will later be analyzed by an algorithm to first identify "silent" symptoms to prevent a progress of the disease-causing symptoms.

The prevention program begins by informing the participant of their current condition. Depending on what has been identified, more movements or support in visiting the correct physician and getting the correct treatment is planned. Additionally, the project also considers people who already have an illness, for example from a stroke, fracture (e.g., caused by osteoporosis), or heart attack. Here, the system will aim to prevent a secondary infection or second disease, or as a fall back in the recovering progress.

REACH is split into four subsystems; sensing and monitoring, analyzing and planning, motivation and intervention, and Personalized Interior Intelligent Units (PI²Us).

5.6.1 Subsystem 1: Sensing and Monitoring

This subsystem involves recording, monitoring, and formatting user-specific physical, physiological, and biometric data followed later by a detailed investigation and analysis. Basic sensors which can be used for this purpose for example include accelerometers, gyroscopes (like the implemented sensors in smartphones), bioelectrical sensors (like ECG, EEG, EMG, etc.), electrochemical sensors (like blood glucose meter), optical sensors (like the pulse oximeter), and temperature sensors (ear thermometer to measure on the tympanic) [183]. As illustrated in Figure 5.39, REACH is a solution that proposes its own innovative sensor systems while still remaining compatible with existing sensing systems and technologies (e.g., FitBit).

Additionally, Figure 5.39 shows the approach of the sensor system. There are mainly two groups of sensor types: stationary (i.e., fixed and/or embedded) and ambulant (i.e., wearable and/or mobile) sensors. The approach of the modularity, as described in Sections 5.2, 5.4, and 5.5, has to be applied especially for the stationary sensor types.

5.6.2 Subsystem 2: Analysis and Planning

The best measurements are worthless if something is not done. Here, subsystem 2 is used to process and analyze the obtained data from Subsystem 1 in order to generate a

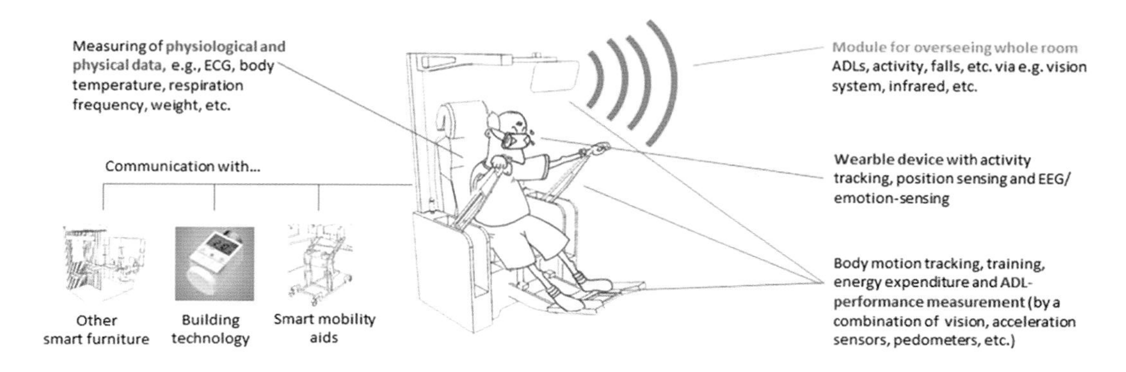

Figure 5.39 Subsystem 1: An example of a stationary furniture implemented with sensor modules that are in communication with wearable sensors so as to capture physiological and physical data of the elderly.

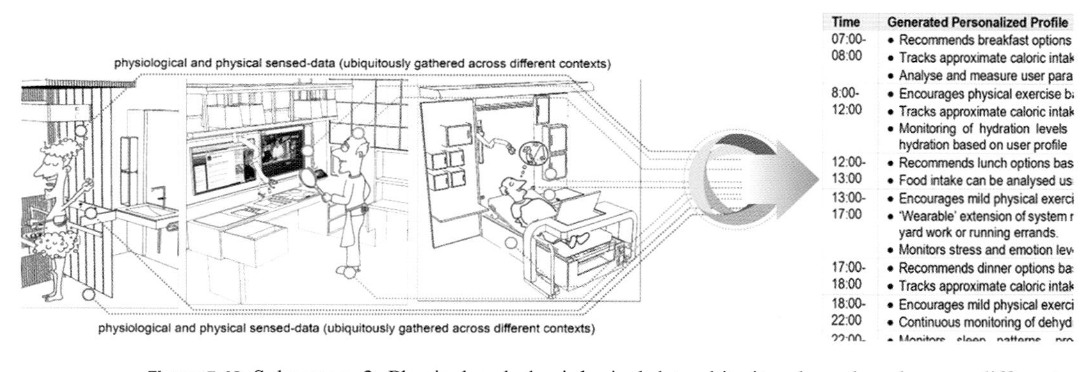

Figure 5.40 Subsystem 2: Physical and physiological data ubiquitously gathered across different contexts and used to generate a personalized regimen.

holistic user profile with personalized motivation and intervention solutions. The algorithm, which will use the input of Subsystem 1, will generate the user profile while considering the user habits, medical history, and lifestyle. Health-related parameters and recommendation strategies will be enabled to promote healthy habits and improve the overall health condition of the elderly, or at least slow down the design progress.

To do so, this subsystem is split into three parts: First, the data reception module receives the collected and forwarded data from Subsystem 1, and second, the analysis module analyzes the data, which consists of machine-learning, data-mining, activity recognition, recommender systems, and statistical analysis processes and methods (see Figure 5.40).

The third module (the planning module) generates the Inter- and Intra-Personal Profiles generated in the previous modules in order to generate admissible action plans for medical experts, patients, and a variety of autonomous systems. These action plans are then delivered in three different outputs, namely Long-term Correlation, Recommendation Strategies, and Disease Prevention Strategies.

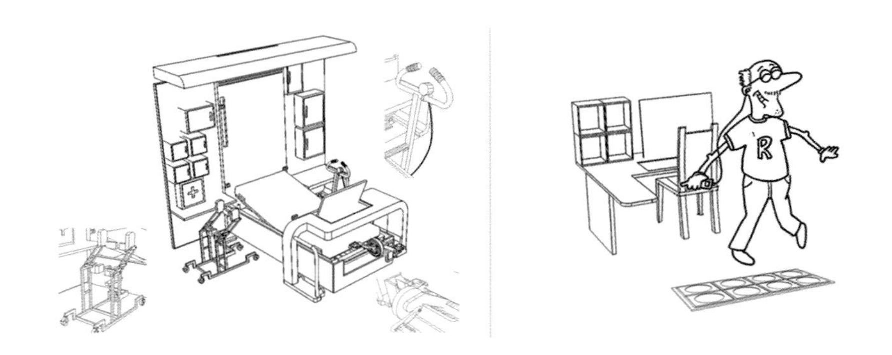

Figure 5.41 Subsystem 3: passive mode interventions for the night (left) and active recommendation intervention for the day-time (right).

5.6.3 Subsystem 3: Motivation and Intervention

This subsystem consists of intervention solutions (i.e., applications, products, and services) which by considering the conclusions ascertained by the analysis and planning processes of subsystem 2 will adapt to the individual needs of the user. Studies suggest that physical intervention devices not only require effectiveness but also motivational strategies because the user may tend to lose interest/motivation in the device [184] [185]. Therefore, REACH designs physical devices embedded with motivational strategies in their schemes and enables effective motivational considerations for day and night (see Figure 5.41).

These intervention solutions focus on the form of applications, devices, and services, and are divided into four main categories:

- Training modules unobtrusively embedded into furniture.
- Mobility- and mobilization-assistance devices, both complementary/supplementary to smart furniture and stand alone.
- Personalized nutrition via limited 3D printing of certain foods to cater for the palate of the user, while managing healthy nutrition.
- Playware to keep the user engaged in a physical and cognitive stimulating way.

In summary, with the guidance of these thematic categories, REACH will provide a variety of products, ranging from furniture-scale to exercise equipment to hand-held playware devices, as well as multifunctional systems for the promotion of activity of all muscle-groups for rehabilitation purposes. Furthermore, the intervention modules have to be designed from beginning on with sophisticated motivation strategies (e.g., suggested by [186]) to keep the user actively stimulated and engaged physically, mentally, and emotionally.

5.6.4 Subsystem 4: Personalized Interior Intelligent Units (PI²Us)

The subsystem of Personalized Interior Intelligent Units (PI²Us) are considered as a type of furniture within the environment (see Figure 5.42). They integrate ambient sensing

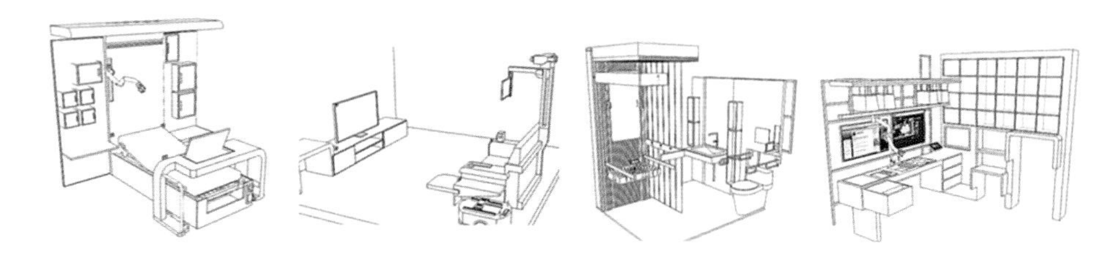

Figure 5.42 Subsystem 4: examples of Personalized Interior Intelligent Units (PI²U).

functions from subsystem 1, and the motivation and intervention modules of subsystem 3 in a manner that enables the use of functionality through one compact element substituting, supplementing, and complementing the existing furniture (e.g., directly implemented into the bed). The PI²Us have to be seamlessly integrated to ensure that technology operates effectively and imperceptibly in the background.

REACH also deals with the optimization of the products architecture and the management of PI²U's complexity through modularity which can be considered a key factor for achieving replicability, mass-production, as well as customization of the PI²Us.

6 Future Trends and Developments

In this chapter, a possible outlook into the future is provided. Considering the newest technology on the market in the young research field of AAL (see Chapter 4), and the youngest research projects (see Chapter 5), new possibilities will exist in the future design of buildings. Buildings mainly consist of four walls and a ceiling, with water and electrical supply. However, with increasing demand for assistive technologies, and with an increasing technology readiness level (TRL) [187] for assistive technologies, there will be a time when this new technology approach will fuse with future building design and construction.

6.1 Robotic and Automated Repair, Renovation, and Maintenance in Other Fields

The techniques and procedures used in other fields could be implemented, after an adaptation, in building renovation and AAL topics. In this chapter, the general ideas behind these fields will be explained.

6.1.1 Aircraft Maintenance Repair Overhaul (MRO)

The main commercial passenger aircrafts fly under extreme circumstances. Often, they are constantly in use and they therefore need constant checking, maintenance, and if needed, repairs. The life span of a plane is often 30 years, and during their lifespan many of their parts are repaired. In order to successfully and efficiently achieve this goal, new technologies have been developed.

For instance, at the Lufthansa Technik AG center [188], three main research concepts have been conceived:

- Adaptive CNC milling: cost-efficient repair processes for the valuable components;
- Robot-based CFRP material repair procedure ready for mobile deployment;
- Augmented Reality.

For instance, within the research project name “CAIRE,” a robot placed in a mobile platform was able to recognize and repair damages on the external fuselage of an airplane.

It has to be said that the repair of the aircraft takes place in a hangar: a controlled environment when compared to other buildings. Also, with regard to logistics, it can be

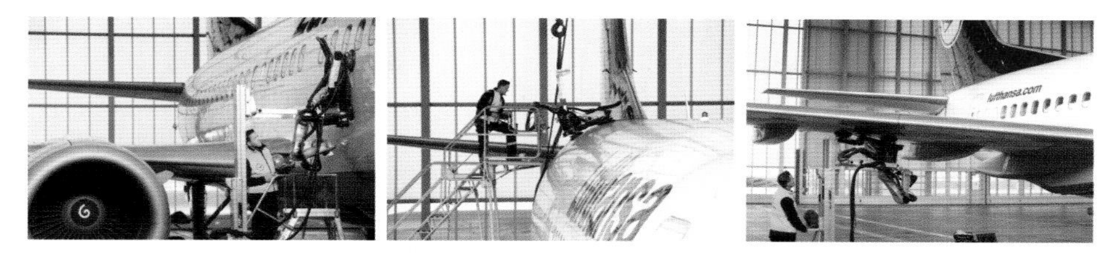

Figure 6.1 Automated detection and repair of composite materials.
Images of the CAIRE project. Lufthansa Technik AG.

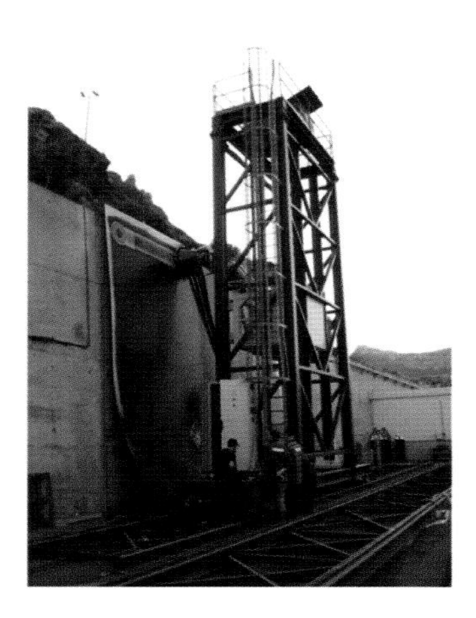

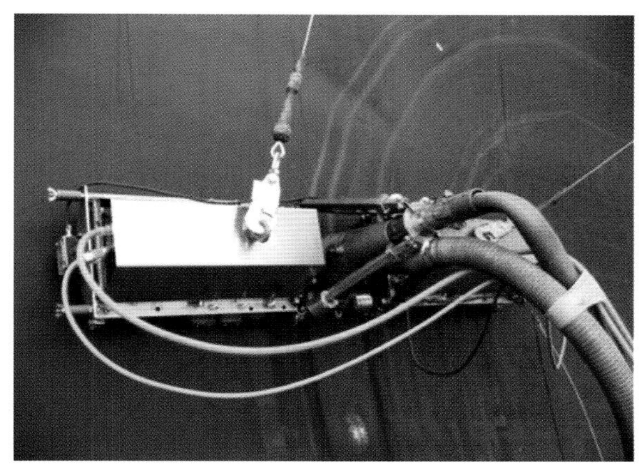

Figure 6.2 Ship bulk repair, by robots; Fernandez-Andrés et al. [189].
Universidad Politécnica de Cartagena (UPCT)

said that the main necessary items for the renovation can either be on the workshop or must arrive on time.

6.1.2 Automated Repair of Ships

The ship industry is similar to the building industry. Regarding maintenance, several robots have already been developed. As with buildings, two aspects must be considered:

- The ship's hull (body)
- The services and mechanical devices.

In regard to the operability of the robots and considering that the repair of the ships is mostly outdoors, there is parallelism with buildings. These concepts are explained further by Fernandez-Andrés et al. [189].

6.1.3 Automated Maintenance, Repair, and Replacement of Oil and Gas Platforms

Oil and gas plants normally consist of kilometers of pipes and tubes which are normally within corrosive environments. Especially for off-shore oil and gas platforms, there is a need to replace damaged elements [190].

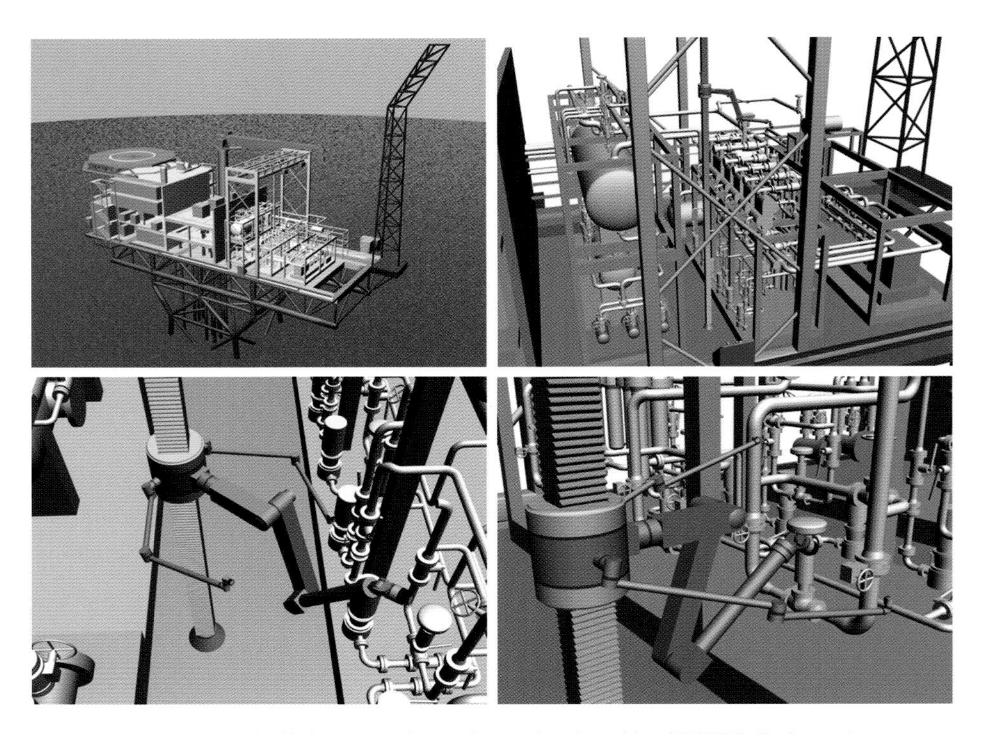

Figure 6.3 Simulation of off-shore robotic platforms developed by SINTEF (Robotnor). Courtesy of Statoil and SINTEF

- In these cases, the replaced elements need to be fixed fast enough in order not to stop the extraction of oil or gas.
- The possibilities of on-site manufacturing are reduced due to the decreased space of the platform. Therefore, already built-in modules are used. These modules are prefabricated in an on-shore factory.

6.1.4 Medical Implant Technology

Medical implants are meant to replace or support damaged biological bodies. Somehow, this concept is very much related to building refurbishment, where the unnecessary, defective, or downgraded building elements need to be removed and replaced. Which knowledge can be subtracted from the field of medical implants and reproduced in building refurbishment? In medical implanting, there is an adaptation and fixation of a "standard element" onto a particular geometry. Similar to the case of the buildings, every biological body has a particular and different geometry, and therefore, data acquisition is particularly of high importance. Besides, the implanting technology takes into consideration that the manual positioning of the implant is itself prone to some tolerances. Focusing on dental implants, three parts can be identified: the implant, the abutment, and the crown. Briefly explained, a dental implant process is as follows:

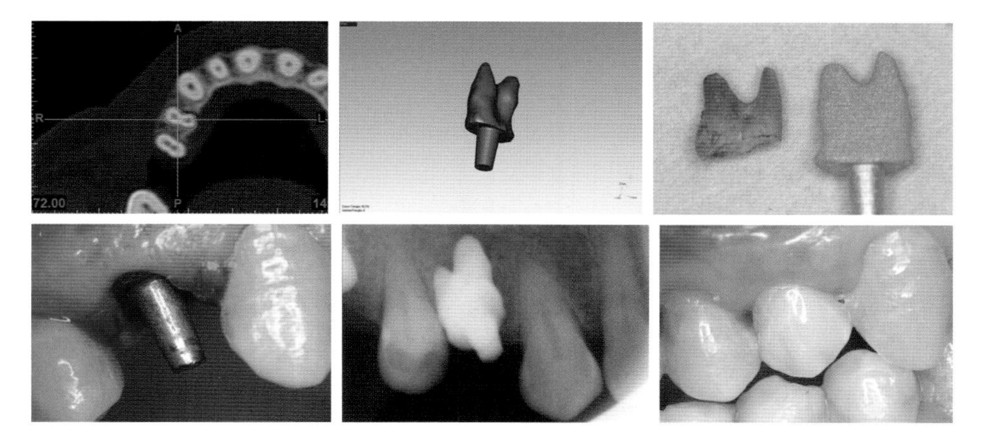

Figure 6.4 Implanting technology. Previous measurement of the teeth, including the root. Create the 3D .stl file for the implant. Insertion of the implant on its required location.
Images by Dr. Mangano [191]

- Session 1: First, there is an overall measurement with X-ray or Computed Tomography (CT) scan. This step is done prior to surgery in order to check the current condition of bones and teeth.
- Session 2: Once there is an accurate diagnosis and the treatment is defined, the surgery process can start:
  - First, a hole is carefully made onto the bone, controlling the location with an alignment pin. After that, the implant is inserted into the hole.
  - Once the implant fixture is inserted into the bone, another geometrical data acquisition is necessary so that the crown can be accurately produced. There are two ways for doing so:
    - Conventional impression taking with flexible material.
    - Digital data scanning. This procedure is more accurate than the conventional impression.
- Normally in a specialized outsourced workshop, the crown is accurately crafted in specialized workshops.
- Session 3: On a final surgery session, the abutment and the crown are inserted.

Recent studies [191] show that there are possibilities to create a bespoke implant that can be placed onto the cavity of the root. This can be done using direct laser metal forming (DLMF) for the manufacturing of the implant, which can also prevent the need of several surgery procedures.

6.1.5 How Can These Concepts Be Adapted onto Building Renovation and Maintenance?

Can these procedures or protocols and technologies be implemented into the building upgrading process? Already, some studies have focused on the possibility of the rearrangement of the final prefabricated module. In our case, however, the question here is if these procedures can be extrapolated to building renovation. In summary, it can be said that in all the analyzed processes, there were some clear emerging concepts. First, there is a measurement of the element to be refurbished. Then, the adjustment of the product and sometimes, a robotic placement. Nevertheless, the robotic installation is a challenge in all cases.

6.2 Future Technological Trends

It is expected that the interconnection of things will also affect the AAL area. Wearables and sensors directly attached to the body, as well as intervention options, will be distributed not only into the furniture and home environment, as depicted in Figure 6.5. Also, neighborhoods, public streets, and even factories will become equipped with AAL technology into their environments, as this is motivated by the need to keep a high life quality for the workforce.

Also, there currently exists no link. An example here is in the car industry; looking back 30 years ago, the car was mainly a mechanical device, but now has assistive systems for safety and comfort unobtrusively embedded in the car, e.g., ABS (antilocking braking system), EBD (electronics brake-force distribution), SRS Air Bags (supplemental restraint system air bags), parking sensors, and cruise control [192]. Furthermore, systems like fatigue detection also exist [193]. The projects as presented in Chapter 5 are aiming to implement the safety and comfort functions through home add-ons; this approach also can be seen in the car industry (e.g., modular navigation systems). Therefore, basic services will probably be implemented in pre-fabricated building modules, resulting in standard assistive functions in apartments or houses of the future.

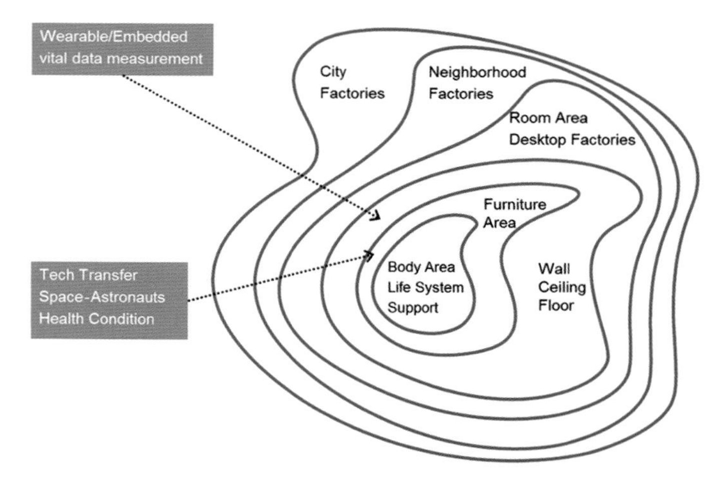

Figure 6.5 Expected networking of things in the future, including the current state of technology and ongoing research.
Source: Thomas Bock

At the moment, for instance, there are ongoing projects which try to develop settlements that produce their own necessary current. This new development of energy harvesting implemented into new buildings provides also the link to indoor (and, maybe later, outdoor) assistance. For example, the project ZERO-PLUS ("Achieving near Zero and Positive Energy Settlements in Europe using Advanced Energy Technology") is developing new designs for high energy–performing buildings. In this project, a modular approach which allows the build-up of zero net energy and providing current to buildings by use of highly efficient insulation, heating, and lighting, as well as by innovative energy production technologies (i.e., Linear Fresnel Reflectors, etc.), is considered [194].

Moreover, the aspect of offsite or prefabrication building modules is investigated by research projects like Building Energy Renovation Through Timber Prefabricated Modules (BERTIM). This project is investigating the opportunity to renovate and improve energy performance while at the same time also improving the air quality, aesthetics, and comfort. Therefore, prefabricated modules that include all necessary water pipes and current wires will be produced. Here, the interfacing of these modules by specially designed connectors as described in [139] is one of the main challenges being solved as part of this project.

Fusing these projects with AAL, e.g., by implementing the assistive AAL technology for safety (e.g., fall detection, as mentioned in Chapter 5), or comfort (assistance in getting clothes on, etc., as described in Chapter 5), would increase the aesthetic and life quality at the same time. Additionally, connecting these modules to plug-and-play modular interfaces (e.g., by using similar connectors as described in [139]) and to a power supply (e.g., a solar cell), which is used in the building (as proposed in ZERO PLUS), can be seen as topics for future research interests of high tech architecture and civil engineers.

6.3 Future Research/Visions for AAL and Construction Automation

The possibilities of AAL technology are not limited to prefabricated modules (e.g., furniture, walls, ceiling, etc., see Figure 6.6), which embed all service functions in modular power generating prefabricated apartment and house modules as described in Chapter 1. Wearables can improve safety on construction sites by predicting outcomes. For example, the EVA suits for space walks are equipped with some wearables (see Section 1.1), which aim to measure the stress levels of astronauts.

Stress levels are of interest because high stress leads to mistakes. Additionally, under prolonged stress, health conditions suffer. Attention is important as a lot of accidents happen when people are distracted. For example, motormen (e.g., in German ICE trains) have to give permanent feedback of their attention to their work, by using a pedal on the chair ground. Through arrhythmic pressure, the motorman gives the train feedback that he is awake and focused. If the motorman stops, or becomes too arrhythmical in the feedback, the train knows that the motorman is not awake or focused and will stop the ride. Following the example of the trains, AAL systems can also be used in the

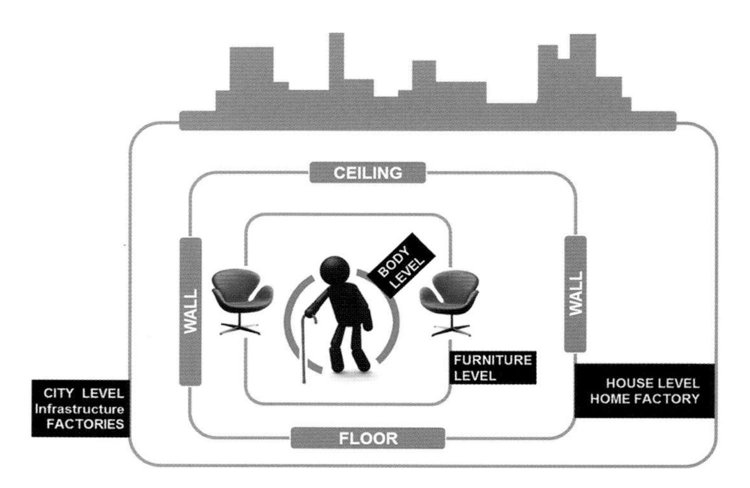

Figure 6.6 Possible prefabrication modules starting on the body level, going to the home environment, and probably even into the city level.
Source: Thomas Bock

construction site to determine the attention and conscious of the workers so as to prevent accidents.

AAL technology, which also focuses on scanning and measuring health parameters like pulse, blood pressure, breath, etc., can help to retrieve similar information from construction workers, which would allow an intervention before an accident happens. Additionally, determination of whether the work conditions and behavior are appropriate to the health condition (ergonomically correct lifting of objects, etc.) can be proved. The ability of a worker can be maintained or kept. This is very important because the number of available workers is decreasing as the population ages (see Section 1.2). Being able to work at construction sites in old age is an exception to what is typical. However, by using AAL technology at the workplaces, especially on such dangerous places like construction sites, these exceptions might change.

In addition, it sounds strange to combine two totally different fields; AAL is a highly interdisciplinary research area while civil engineering and architecture are the exact opposite. Nevertheless, fusing two different fields always results in new possibilities and new interdisciplinary solutions, which will improve the quality of life and work. For example, mechatronics is the fusion of electronics and mechanics. Later on, medicine and mechatronics were fused into medical engineering. The fusion of these three different engineering fields resulted in a myriad of medical devices. Robotics and AAL are a multidisciplinary fusion of even more scientific fields (electrotechnology, mechanics, informatics, medicine, regulation technology, social sciences, etc.) and its promises are already showing great potential.

However, the possibilities created by fusing AAL with civil engineering and high-tech architecture is at the moment unpredictable but allows for high expectations for cities of the future. Table 6.1 gathers all the robotic ambience categories and systems mentioned in this book.

Table 6.1 Robotic ambience categories and systems.

Category	Category	Subsystems	Planning components/scope
Physical	Classical 'passive' subsystems	Building structure	Bearing structure: steel concrete, brickwork etc.
		Building infrastructure	Water pipes, cables, air circulation, energy generating modules etc.
		Building modules	Walls, columns, windows, doors, ceiling etc.
		Surfaces	Painting, stucco, plastering, textures etc.
Digital	Emerging 'active' subsystem	Mechatronic systems	Wall cabinet lift, worktop unit lift, kitchen appliance lift, liftable toilet
		Embedded micro systems	Sensors, actors: sensor floor, heat sensors etc., sensors for health conditions
		Wearable/implanted devices	Sensors, actors in the body area, sensor shirts, implanted sensors/actors
		Intelligent appliances	Controllable lights, refrigerator, washing machine
		Interfaces	Touch screens, voicemail, communication devices, mobile phones
		Robotics	E.g. Robotic Bed by Panasonic
		Mobility systems	Intelligent wheelchairs, Toyota i-Swing, Toyota i-unit, HAL Cyberdyne
		ICT-enables applications	ICT platforms, monitoring/tracking systems, ambient intelligence, pro-activity
		Physical and digital services	Care services, supply with goods, supply with information, emergency alert/call etc.

Source: Thomas Bock

References

[1] T. Bock, "A Concept for a Building System with Integrated Service Robot Technology," in *Proceedings of the Dai San Kenchiku Seko Robot Symposium, S.7–10, S.19–22*, Tokyo, 1989.

[2] T. Von Zglinicki, "Alter und Altern," in *Physiologie des Menschen mit Pathophysiologie*, Berlin Heidelberg: Springer, 2010, pp. 877–891.

[3] C. Darwin, *On the Origin of Species by Means of Natural Selection. 1859*, Toronto: Broadview, 2003.

[4] M. C. Carter, V. J. Burley, C. Nykjaer, and J. E. Cade, "Adherence to a Smartphone Application for Weight Loss Compared to Website and Paper Diary: Pilot Randomized Controlled Trial," *Journal of Medical Internet Research*, Vol. 15, No. 4, 2013.

[5] J. Tran, R. Tran, and J. White, "Smartphone-Based Glucose Monitors and Applications in the Management of Diabetes: An Overview of 10 Salient 'Apps' and a Novel Smartphone-Connected Blood Glucose Monitor," *Clinical Diabetes*, Vol. 30, No. 4, pp. 173–178, 2012.

[6] D.-Y. Fei and X. Zhao, "A Biomedical Sensor System for Real-Time Monitoring of Astronauts' Physiological Parameters during Extra-Vehicular Activities," *Computers in Biology and Medicine*, Vol. 40, No. 7, pp. 635–642, 2010.

[7] P. Rashidi, "A Survey on Ambient-Assisted Living Tools for Older Adults," *IEEE Journal of Biomedical and Health Informatics*, Vol. 17, No. 3, pp. 579–590, 2013.

[8] J. M. Eklund, T. R. Hansen, S. Jonathan, and S. Shankar, "Information Technology for Assisted Living at Home: Building a Wireless Infrastructure for Assisted Living," in *IEEE Engineering in Medicine and Biology 27th Annual Conference*, Shanghai: IEEE, 2005.

[9] S. Dubowsky, F. Genot, S. Godding, H. Kozono, A. Skwersky, H. Yu, and L. S. Yu, "PAMM – A Robotic Aid to the Elderly for Mobility Assistance and Monitoring: A 'Helping-Hand' for the Elderly," in *International Conference on Robotics & Automation*, San Francisco, CA, 2000.

[10] F. Vetere, H. Davis, M. Gibbs, and S. Howard, "The Magic Box and Collage: Responding to the Challenge of Distributed Intergenerational Play," *International Journal of Human-Computer Studies*, Vol. 67, No. 2, pp. 165–178, 2009.

[11] C.-A. Smarr, C. B. Fausset, and W. A. Rogers, "Understanding the Potential for Robot Assistance for Older Adults in the Home Environment," School of Psychology, Human Factors and Aging Laboratory, Georgia Inst. Technology, Atlanta, 2011.

[12] B. Graf, U. Reiser, M. Hägele, K. Mauz, and P. Klein, "Robotic Home Assistant Care-O-bot® 3: Product Vision and Innovation Platform," in *IEEE Workshop on Advanced Robotics and its Social Inpacts*, Tokyo, Japan, 2009.

[13] T. Mukai, S. Hirano, H. Nakashima, Y. Kato, Y. Sakaida, G. Shijie, and S. Hosoe, "Development of a Nursing-Care Assistant Robot RIBA That Can Lift a Human in Its

Arms," in *IEEE/RSJ International Conference on Intelligent Robots and Systems*, Taipei, Taiwan, 2010.
[14] Z. Xu, T. Deyle, and C. C. Kemp, "1000 Trails: An Empirically Validated End Effector That Robustly Grasps Objects from the Floor," in *IEEE International Conference on Robotics and Automation*, Kobe, Japan, 2009.
[15] T. Mukai, S. Hirano, H. Nakashima, Y. Kato, Y. Sakaida, S. Guo, and S. Hosoe, "Development of a Nursing-Care Assistant Robot RIBA That Can Lift a Human in Its Arms," in *IEEE/RSJ International Conference on Intelligent Robots and Systems*, Taipei, Taiwan, 2010.
[16] P. Rashidi, "Keeping the Resident in the Loop: Adapting the Smart Home to the User," *IEEE Transactions on Systems, Man, and Cybernetics-Part A: Systems and Humans*, Vol. 39, No. 5, pp. 949–959, 2009.
[17] N. Batini, T. Callen, and W. McKibbin, "The Global Impact of Demographic Change," IMF Working Paper, 2006.
[18] J. A. Kolmer and B. Lucke, "A Study of the Histologic Changes Produced Experimentally in Rabbits by Arsphenamin," *Archives of Dermatology and Syphilology*, Vol. 3, No. 4, pp. 483–514, 1921.
[19] W. Burckhardt, "Die Penicillinbehandlung der Syphilis," *Dermatology*, Vol. 99, No. 5, pp. 286–296, 1949.
[20] O. Pötzsch and F. Rößger, "Demographic Analyses, Methods and Projections, Births and Deaths" Section, "Germany's population by 2060, Results of the 13th Coordinated Population Projection," Statistisches Bundesamt, Wiesbaden, 2015.
[21] T. Champion and J. Shepherd, "Demographic Change in Rural England," *In The Ageing Countryside: The Growing Older Population of Rural England,* pp. 29–50, 2006.
[22] K. Geppert and M. Gorning, "Mehr Jobs, mehr Menschen: Die Anziehungskraft der großen Städte wächst," *DIW-Wochenbericht,* No. 19, pp. 2–10, 2010.
[23] M. Decker, "Ein Abbild des Menschen: Humanoide Roboter," in *Inofmation und Menschenbild*, Berlin Heidelberg: Springer, 2010, pp. 41–62.
[24] C. Bartneck, T. Nomura, T. Kanda, T. Suzuki, and K. Kensuke, "A cross-cultural study on attitudes towards robots," *HCI international,* 2005.
[25] J. Cameron, Regisseur, *The Terminator*. [Film]. USA, UK: MGM, 1984.
[26] P. Chung, A. R. Jones, Y. Kawajiri, T. Koike, M. Maeda, K. Morimoto, and S. Watanabe, Regisseure, *The Animatrix*. [Film]. USA, Japan: Silver, Joel, 2003.
[27] J. L. Jones, "Robots at the Tipping Point," *The Road to the IRobot Roomba*, Vol. 13, No. 1, pp. 76–78, 2006.
[28] A. Wißnet, *Roboter in Japan*, München: Iudicium-Verlag, 2007.
[29] "Kouka-ninjya museum," Kouka Ninya, [Online]. Available: www.kouka-ninjya.com/. [Zugriff am 17 August 2018].
[30] "Izushi Kabuki Theatre," Toyooka City, [Online]. Available: https://visitkinosaki.com/explore/things-to-see/izushi-kabuki-theatre/. [Zugriff am 23 November 2017].
[31] T. Linner, W. Pan, C. Georgoulas, B. Georgescu, J. Güttler, and T. Bock, "Co-adaptation of Robot Systems, Processes and In-house Environments for Professional Care Assistance in an Ageing Society," *Procedia Engineering*, Vol. 85, pp. 328–338, 2014.
[32] T. Bock, *A Study on Robot-Oriented Construction and Building System*, Tokyo: University of Tokyo, 1989.
[33] H. R. D'Allemagne, *Histoire des Jouets*, Paris: Libraire Hachette & Cie. , 1902.
[34] "Bandai," [Online]. Available: www.bandai.co.jp/. [Zugriff am 03 09 2018].

[35] S. Intille, "A New Research Challenge: Persuasive Technology to Motivate Healthy Aging," *IEEE Transactions on Information Technology in Biomedicine*, Vol. 8, No. 3, pp. 235–237, 2004.

[36] H. Maier, *Supercentenarians*, London: Springer, 2010.

[37] E. Aarts, H. Harwig, and M. Schuurmans, *Ambient Intelligence: The Invisible Future*, New York: McGraw-Hill, 2001.

[38] R. Want, "An Introduction to RFID Technology," *IEEE Pervasive Computing*, vol. 5, no. 1, pp. 25–33, 2006.

[39] T. Linner, C. Georgoulas, and T. Bock, "Advanced Building Engineering: Deploying Mechatronics and Robotics in Architecture," *Geronntechnology*, Vol. 11, No. 2, p. 8, 2012.

[40] H. Hauner, "Managing Type 2 Diabetes Mellitus in Patients with Obesity," *Treatments in Endocrinology*, Vol. 3, No. 4, pp. 223–232, 2004.

[41] World Health Organization, "Pulse Oximetry Training Manual," *WHO Library Cataloguing-in-Publication Data*, Geneva, 2011.

[42] Measurment Specialities, *Detector Assembly EPM-4001,* 2014.

[43] Burr-Brown Products from Texas Instruments, *Precision, Low Power, 18MHz Transimpedance Amplifier, OPA 381, OPA 2381*, Texas Instruments Incorporated, 2004.

[44] S. Prahl, "Tabulated Molar Extinction Coefficient for Hemoglobin in Water," *Oregon Medical Laser Center,* No. 4, 1998.

[45] A. Roguin, "Scipione Riva-Rocci and the Men behind the Mercury Sphygmomanometer," *International Journal of Clinical Practice*, Vol. 60, No. 1, pp. 73–79, 2006.

[46] D. Chungcharoen, "Genesis of Korotkoff Sounds," *American Journal of Physiology*, Vol. 270, No. 1, pp. 190–194, 1964.

[47] R. Brandes and R. Busse, "Kreislauf," in *Physiologie des Menschen mit Pathophysiologie*, Heidelberg, Springer Medizin, 2010, pp. 572–626.

[48] P. A. Mackowiak, "Physiological Rationale for Suppression of Fever," *Oxford Journals, Medicine & Health, Clinical Infectious Diseases*, Vol. 31, No. 5, pp. 185–189, 200.

[49] P. Persson, "Energie- und Wärmehaushalt, Thermoregulation," in *Physiologie des Menschen*, Berlin Heidelberg, Springer, 2010, pp. 834–853.

[50] P. Perera, M. Fernando, S. Maththananda, and R. Samaranayake, "Accuracy of Measuring Axillary Temperature Using Mercury in Glass Thermometers in Children under Five Years: A Cross Sectional Observational Study," *Health*, Vol. 6, No. 16, pp. 2115–2120, 2014.

[51] J.-Y. Lefrant, L. Muller, J. Emmanuel de La Coussaye, M. Benbabaali, C. Lebris, N. Zeitoun, C. Mari, G. Saïssi, and J. Ripart, "Temperature Measurement in Intensive Care Patients: Comparison of Urinary Bladder, Oesophageal, Rectal, Axillary, and Inguinal Methods versus Pulmonary Artery Core Method," *Intensive Care Medicine*, Vol. 29, No. 3, pp. 414–418, 2003.

[52] A. S. El-Radhi and S. Patel, "An Evaluation of Tympanic Thermometry in a Paediatric Emergency Department," *Emergency Medicine Journal*, Vol. 23, No. 1, pp. 40–41, 2006.

[53] S. Smitz, T. Giagoultsis, W. Dewé, and A. Albert, "Comparison of Rectal and Infrared Ear Temperatures in Older Hospital Inpatients," *Journal of the American Geriatrics Society*, Vol. 48, No. 1, pp. 63–66, 2015.

[54] G. I. Gasim, I. R. Musa, M. T. Abdien, and A. Ishag, "Accuracy of Tympanic Temperature Measurement Using an Infrared Tympanic Membrane Thermometer," *BMC research notes*, Vol. 6, No. 1, 2013.

[55] M. Dettenkofer und F. Daschner, "Prävention von Infektionen in der," in *Praktische Krankenhaushygiene und Umweltschutz*, Berlin Heidelberg, Springer, 1997, pp. 503–518.

[56] C.-C. Liu, R.-E. Chang, and W.-C. Chang, "Limitations of Forehead Infrared Body Temperature Detection for Fever Screening for Severe Acute Respiratory Syndrome," *Infection Control & Hospital Epidemiology*, Vol. 25, No. 12, pp. 1109–1111, 2004.

[57] J. A. Kistemaker, E. A. Den Hartog, and H. A. M. Daanen, "Reliability of an Infrared Forehead Skin Thermometer for Core Temperature Measurements," *Journal of Medical Engineering & Technology*, Vol. 30, No. 4, pp. 252–261, 2006.

[58] R. F. Grais, J. H. Ellis, and G. E. Glass, "Assessing the Impact of Airline Travel on the Geographic Spread of Pandemic Influenza," *European Journal of Epidemiology*, Vol. 18, No. 11, pp. 1065–1072, 2003.

[59] L. Simonsen, M. J. Clarke, L. B. Schonberger, N. H. Arden, N. J. Cox, and K. Fukuda, "Pandemic versus Epidemic Influenza Mortality: A Pattern of Changing Age Distribution," *Journal of Infectious Diseases*, Vol. 178, No. 1, pp. 53–60, 1998.

[60] H. Nishiura and K. Kamiya, "Fever Screening during the Influenza (H1N1–2009) Pandemic at Narita International Airport, Japan," *BMC infectious diseases*, Vol. 11, No. 1, 2011.

[61] E. F. J. Ring, A. Jung, J. Zuber, P. Rutowski, B. Kalicki, and U. Bajwa, "Detecting Fever in Polish Children by Infrared Thermography," *Proceedings of the 9th International Conference on Quantitative Infrared Thermography*, Vol. 2, No. 5, 2008.

[62] A. V. Nguyen, N. J. Cohen, H. Lipman, C. M. Brown, N.-A. Molinari, W. L. Jackson, H. L. Kirking, P. Szymanowski, T. W. Wilson, B. A. Salhi, R. R. Roberts, D. W. Stryker, and D. B. Fishbein, "Comparison of 3 Infrared Thermal Detection Systems and Self-Report for Mass Fever Screening," *Emerging Infectious Diseases*, Vol. 16, No. 11, pp. 1710–1717, 2010.

[63] L.-S. Chan, G. T. Y. Cheung, I. J. Lauder, and C. R. Kumana, "Screening for Fever by Remote-Sensing Infrared Thermographic Camera," *Travel Medicine*, Vol. 11, No. 5, pp. 273–279, 2004.

[64] B. B. Lowell and G. I. Shulman, "Mitochondrial Dysfunction and Type 2 Diabetes," *Science*, Vol. 307, No. 5708, pp. 384–387, 2005.

[65] T. Kriegel and W. Schellenberger, "Enzyme in Forschung, Diagnostik und Therapie," in *Löffler/Petrides Biochemie und Pathobiochemie*, Berlin Heidelberg, Springer, 2014, pp. 125–129.

[66] W. Einthoven, G. Fahr, and A. de Waart, "Über die Richtung und die manifste Grösse der Potentialschwankungen im menschlichen Herzen und über den Einfluss der herzlage auf die Form des Elektrokardiogramms," *Pflügers Archiv European Journal of Physiology*, Vol. 150, No. 6, pp. 275–315, 1913.

[67] H. M. Piper, "Herzerregung," in *Physiologie des Menschen mit Pathophysiologie*, Berlin Heidelberg, Springer, 2010, pp. 517–538.

[68] W. Nehb, "Zur Standardisierung der Brustwand-Ableitungen des Elektrokardiogramms," *Journal of Molecular Medicine*, Vol. 17, No. 51, pp. 1807–1811, 1938.

[69] C. Fleischer, C. Reinicke and G. Hommel, "Predicting the Intended Motion with EMG Signals for an Exoskeleton Orthosis Controller," in *IEEE/RSJ International Conference on Intelligent Robots and Systems*, 2005.

[70] M. Mulas, M. Folgheraiter, and G. G., "An EMG-Controlled Exoskeleton for Hand Rehabilitation," in *9th International Conference on Rehabilitation Robotics*, 2005.

[71] N. Birbaumer and R. F. Schmidt, "Wach-Schlaf-Rhythmus und Aufmerksamkeit," in *Physiologie des Menschen mit Pathophysiologie*, Berlin Heidelberg, Springer, 2010, pp. 181–200.

[72] N. M. Kaplan, "The Deadly Quartet: Upper-Body Obesity, Glucose Intolerance, Hypertriglyceridemia, and Hypertension," *Archives of Internal Medicine*, Vol. 149, No. 7, pp. 1514–1520, 1989.

[73] S. C. Bundrick, M. S. Thearle, C. A. Venti, J. Krakoff, and S. Votruba, "Soda Consumption during Ad Libitum Food Intake Predicts Weight Change," *Journal of the Academy of Nutrition and Dietetics*, Vol. 114, No. 3, pp. 444–449, 2014.

[74] J. Stern, A. S. Grant, C. A. Thomson, L. Tinker, L. Hale, K. Brennan, N. Woods, and Z. Chen, "Short Sleep Duration Is Associated with Decreased Serum Leptin, Increased Energy Intake, and Decreased Diet Quality in Postmenopausal Women," *Obesity*, Vol. 22, No. 5, pp. E55-E61, 2014.

[75] K. Ouriel, "Peripheral Arterial Disease," *The Lancet*, Vol. 358, No. 9289, pp. 1257–1264, 2001.

[76] A. Ochsner, J. L. Ochsner, and H. Sanders, "Prevention of Pulmonary Embolism by Caval Ligation," *Annals of Surgery*, Vol. 171, No. 6, pp. 923–936, 1970.

[77] K. M. Anderson, P. M. Odell, P. W. F. Wilson, and W. B. Kannel, "Cardiovascular Disease Risk Profiles," *American Heart Journal*, Vol. 121, No. 1, pp. 293–298, 1991.

[78] G. Donnan, M. Fisher, M. Macleod, and S. Davis, "Stroke," *The Lancet*, Vol. 371, No. 9624, pp. 1612–1623, 2008.

[79] Statistisches Bundesamt, "Sterbefälle für die 10 häufigsten Todesursachen," Statistisches Bundesamt, Wiesbaden, 2014. [Online]. Available: www.destatis.de/DE/ZahlenFakten/GesellschaftStaat/Gesundheit/Todesursachen/Tabellen/HaeufigsteTodesursachen.html;jsessionid=F2CAB274A9559E7F0EA192DE07E10F85.cae3. [Zugriff am 28 07 2016].

[80] J. Marx, "Unraveling the Causes of Diabetes," *Science*, Vol. 296, No. 5568, pp. 686–689, 2002.

[81] G. Herold, *Innere Medizin-Ausgabe 2014*, Kandern: Herold Verlag, 2014.

[82] J. P. Brown and R. G. Josse, "2002 Clinical Practice Guidelines for the Diagnosis and Management of Osteoporosis in Canada," *Canadian Medical Association Journal*, Vol. 167, No. 10, pp. S1-S34, 2002.

[83] J. Iwamoto, T. Takeda, and Y. Sato, "Interventions to Prevent Bone Loss in Astronauts during Space Flight," *The Keio Journal of Medicine*, Vol. 54, No. 2, pp. 55–59, 2005.

[84] B. L. Riggs, J. Jowsey, P. J. Kelly, J. D. Jones, and F. T. Maher, "Effect of Sex Hormones on Bone in Primary Osteoporosis," *Journal of Clinical Investigation*, Vol. 48, No. 6, pp. 1065–1072, 1969.

[85] E. Seeman, L. Melton, W. O'Fallon, and B. Riggs, "Risk Factors for Spinal Osteoporosis in Men," *The American Journal of Medicine*, Vol. 75, No. 6, pp. 977–983, 1983.

[86] A. Schrag, A. Hovris, D. Morley, N. Quinn, and M. Jahanshahi, "Young- versus Older-Onset Parkinson's Disease: Impact of Disease and Psychosocial Consequences," *Movement Disorders*, Vol. 18, No. 11, pp. 1250–1256, 2003.

[87] J. Jankovic, "Parkinson's Disease: Clinical Features and Diagnosis," *Journal of Neurology, Neurosurgery & Psychiatry*, Vol. 79, No. 4, pp. 368–376, 2008.

[88] F. Lehmannn-Horn, "Motorische Systeme," in *Physiologie des Menschen mit Pathophysiologie*, Berlin, Heidelberg, Springer, 2010, pp. 128–162.

[89] M. West, P. D. Coleman, D. G. Flood, and J. C. Troncoso, "Difference in the Pattern of Hippocampal Neuronal Loss in Normal Ageing and Alzheimer's Disease," *The Lancet*, Vol. 344, No. 8925, pp. 769–772, 1994.

[90] N. Bribaumer and R. Schmidt, "Lernen und Gedächtnis," in *Physiologie des Menschen mit Pathophysiologie*, Heidelberg, Berlin, Springer, 2010, pp. 201–217.

[91] P. Mölsä, R. Marttila, and U. Rinne, "Survival and Cause of Death in Alzheimer's Disease and Multi-Infarct Dementia," *Acta Neurologica Scandinavica*, Vol. 74, No. 2, pp. 103–107, 1986.
[92] U. Eysel, "Sehen und Augenbewegungen," in *Phsiologie des Menschen mit Pathophysiologie*, Berlin, Heidelberg, Springer, 2010, pp. 345–385.
[93] P. Grimes and L. von Sallmann, "Lens Epithelium Proliferation in Sugar Cataracts," *Investigative Ophthalmology & Visual Science*, Vol. 7, No. 5, pp. 535–543, 1968.
[94] H. A. Quigley, "Number of People with Glaucoma Worldwide," *British Journal of Ophthalmology*, Vol. 80, pp. 389–393, 1996.
[95] G. Landa, E. Su, P. M. T. Garcia, W. H. Seiple, and R. B. Rosen, "Inner Segment-Outer Segment Junctional Layer Integrity and Corresponding Retinal Sensitivity in Dry and Wet Forms of Age-Related Macular Degeneration," *Retina*, Vol. 31, No. 2, pp. 364–370, 2011.
[96] S. Takeda, I. Morioka, K. Miyshita, A. Okumura, Y. Yoshida, and K. Matsumoto, "Age Variation in the Upper Limit of Hearing," *European Journal of Applied Physiology*, Vol. 65, No. 5, pp. 403–408, 1992.
[97] H.-P. Zenner, "Die Kommunikation des Menschen: Hören und Sprechen," in *Physiologie des Menschen mit Pathophysiologie*, Heidelberg, Springer Medizin, 2010, pp. 316–335.
[98] N. W. D. Mankiw, "The Baby Boom, the Baby Bust, and the Housing Market," *Regional Science and Urban Economics*, Vol. 19, No. 2, pp. 235–258, 1989.
[99] V. Regnier, *Design for Assisted Living: Guidelines for Housing the Physically and Mentally Frail*, London, John Wiley & Sons, 2003.
[100] G. P. D. e. Andrews, *Ageing and Place*, London, Routledge, 2004.
[101] K. W. G. Addae-Dapaah, "Housing and the Elderly in Singapore: Financial and Quality of Life Implications of Ageing in Place," *Journal of Housing and the Built Environment*, Vol. 16, No. 2, pp. 153–178, 2001.
[102] M. Beyeler, Weiterbauen. Wohneigentum im Alter neu nutzen, Basel: Christoph Merian Verlag, 2010.
[103] N. H. U. Kohler, "The Building Stock as a Research Object," *Building Research & Information*, Vol. 30, No. 4, pp. 226–236, 2002.
[104] A. Power, "Does Demolition or Refurbishment of Old and Inefficient Homes Help to Increase Our Environmental, Social and Economic Viability?," *Energy Policy*, Vol. 36, No. 12, pp. 4487–4501, 2008.
[105] https://ec.europa.eu/energy/en/topics/energy-efficiency/buildings, European Commission. [Online]. [Zugriff am 12 June 2017].
[106] www.zenn-fp7.eu, [Online]. [Accessed 11 June 2017].
[107] S. Kose, "Housing Elderly People in Japan," *Ageing International*, Vol. 23, No. 3, pp. 148–164, 1997.
[108] J. Ravetz, "State of the Stock: What Do We Know about Existing Buildings and their Future Prospects?," *Energy Policy*, Vol. 36, No. 12, pp. 4462–4470, 2008.
[109] C. Laura L., "Selectivity Theory: Social Activity in Life-Span Context," *Annual Review of Gerontology and Geriatrics*, Vol. 11, No. 1, pp. 195–217, 1991.
[110] L. Schellen, W. D. van Marken Lichtenbelt, M. G. L. C. Loomans, J. Toftum, and M. H. De Wit, "Differences between Young Adults and Elderly in Thermal Comfort, Productivity, and Thermal Physiology in Response to a Moderate Temperature Drift and a Steady-State Condition," *Indoor Air*, Vol. 20, No. 4, pp. 273–283, 2010.
[111] www.realvalueproject.com/, [Online]. [Zugriff am 12 June 2017].
[112] www.encompass-project.eu/, [Online]. [Zugriff am 12 June 2017].

[113] S. B. B. a. H. M. ,. 1. p.-8. Stansfeld, "Noise and Health in the Urban Environment.," *Reviews on Environmental Health*, Vol. 15, No. 1/2, pp. 43–82, 2000.
[114] D. Y. S. a. L. K. Lo, "Design for Noise Mitigation Measures for Public Housing Developments in Hong Kong," *INTER-NOISE and NOISE-CON Congress and Conference Proceedings*, Vol. 249, No. 4, pp. 3423–3430, 2014, October.
[115] "Noise Simulation and Prediction Software," Noise 3D, [Online]. Available: www.noise3d.com/wordpress/home/#. [Zugriff am 12 June 2017].
[116] V. Tazian, "Lightweight, Flexible, Moldable Acoustic Barrier and Composites Including the Same." U.S. Patent Application Patent 12/560,255., 2009.
[117] "Egoin," Egoin, [Online]. Available: http://egoin.com/. [Zugriff am 12 June 2017].
[118] "People´s Architecture," [Online]. Available: www.peoples-architecture.com/pao/. [Zugriff am 12 June 2017].
[119] J. C. Chung and C. K. Lai, "Snoezelen for Dementia," *Cochrane Database Syst Rev*, Vol. 4, 2002.
[120] U. U., Light and Taste: Third Plane Side-View Combined with Complex Fenestration System Atmospheres under Midday Clear Sky at Restaurants, UPCommons, 2016.
[121] A. Kolanowski, "Restlessness in the Elderly: The Effect of Artificial Lighting," *Nursing Research*, Vol. 39, No. 3, pp. 181–183, 1990.
[122] M. De Rooij, *PhD Dissertation: Arquitectura ante cambios demográficos: la vivienda existente para gente mayor*, Universitat Politècnica de Catalunya, 2014.
[123] "Transformation de la Tour Bois le Prêtre," [Online]. Available: www.lacatonvassal.com/index.php?idp=56. [Zugriff am 12 June 2017].
[124] D. Armstrong, "A Survey of Community Gardens in Upstate New York: Implications for Health Promotion and Community Development," *Health & Place*, Vol. 6, No. 4, pp. 319–327, 2000.
[125] "CATCH – Cucumber Gathering – Green Field Experiments," [Online]. Available: http://echord.eu/catch/. [Zugriff am 12 June 2017].
[126] N. Labonnote, A. Rønnquist, B. Manum, and P. Rüthera, "Additive Construction: State-of-the-Art, Challenges and Opportunities," *Automation in Construction*, Vol. 72, pp. 347–366, 2016.
[127] "Sekisui Owner," Sekisui Chemical Co., Ltd, [Online]. Available: www.sekisuiheim-owner.jp/. [Zugriff am 12 June 2017].
[128] T. L. T. Bock, *Robotic Industrialization: Automation and Robotic Technologies for Customized Component, Module, and Building Prefabrication*, Cambridge, Cambridge University Press, 2015.
[129] S. T. J. Kendall, *Residential Open Building*, London, Routledge, 2010.
[130] N. Suh, *Axiomatic Design: Advances and Applications*, Oxford, The Oxford Series on Advanced Manufacturing, 2001.
[131] CIB W104, [Online]. Available: www.open-building.org/ob/next21.html. [Zugriff am 12 June 2017].
[132] F. Rojo Perez, G. Fernandez-Mayoralas Fernandez, E. Pozo Rivera, and J. M. Rojo Abuin, "Ageing in Place: Predictors of the Residential Satisfaction of Elderly," *Social Indicators Research*, Vol. 54, No. 2, pp. 173–208, 2001.
[133] J. Mankins, "Technology Readiness Levels," *White Paper*, Vol. 6, No. 6, p. 1995, 1995.
[134] A. Kaklauskas, E. K. Zavadskas, S. Raslanas, R. Ginevicius, A. Komka, and P Malinauskas, "Selection of Low-e Windows in Retrofit of Public Buildings by Applying Multiple

Criteria Method COPRAS: A Lithuanian Case," *Energy and Buildings*, Vol. 38, No. 5, pp. 454–462, 2006.

[135] K. K. N. Ishida, "A Study on the Optimization Method for Panel Layout Problem in Drywall," in *Proceedings of the 28th ISARC*, Seoul, Korea, 2011.

[136] F. Bosché, M. Ahmed, Y. Turkan, C. T. Haas, and R. Haas, "The Value of Integrating Scan-to-BIM and Scan-vs-BIM Techniques for Construction Monitoring Using Laser Scanning and BIM: The Case of Cylindrical MEP Components," *Automation in Construction*, Vol. 49, pp. 201–2013, 2015.

[137] E. Lublasser, L. Hildebrand, A. Vollpracht, and S. Brell-Cokcan, "Robot Assisted Deconstruction of Multi-Layered Façade Constructions on the Example of External Thermal Insulation Composite Systems," *Construction Robotics*, pp.1–9, 2017.

[138] "BERTIM project," [Online]. Available: www.bertim.eu. [Zugriff am 12 June 2017].

[139] K. Iturralde, T. Linner, and T. Bock, "Development of a Modular and Integrated Product-Manufacturing-Installation System Kit for the Automation of the Refurbishment Process in the Research Project BERTIM," in *33rd International Symposium on Automation and Robotics in Construction*, Auburn, Alabama, USA, 2016.

[140] "SME Robotics project," [Online]. Available: www.smerobotics.org/demonstrations/d2.html. [Zugriff am 12 June 2017].

[141] "Hephaestus Project," [Online]. Available: www.hephaestus-project.eu/. [Zugriff am 12 June 2017].

[142] United Nations, *World Urbanization Prospects: The 2014 Revision*, New York, United Nations, 2015.

[143] M. Golia, *Cairo: City of Sand*, Cairo, The American University in Cairo Press, 2008.

[144] R. Hu, T. Linner, C. Follini, W. Pan, and T. Bock, "An Affordable and Adaptable Building System to Transform Informal Settlements in Cairo," in *Proceedings of S.ARCH Conference 2018*, Venice, Italy, 2018.

[145] I. Sommerville, *Software Engineering*, Boston, MA, USA, Pearson, 2011.

[146] S. R. a. J. Robertson, *Mastering the Requirements Process*, Upper Saddle River, NJ, USA, Addison-Wesley, 2006.

[147] Y. Cuperus, "An Introduction to Open Building," in *Proceedings of the 9th Annual Conference of the International Group for Lean Construction (IGLC 2001)*, Singapore, 2001.

[148] R. Hu, C. Follini, W. Pan, T. Linner, and T. Bock, "A Case Study on Regenerating Informal Settlements in Cairo using Affordable and Adaptable Building System," *Procedia Engineering*, *Vol. 196*, pp. 113–120, June 2017.

[149] T. Linner, J. Güttler, C. Georgoulas, A. Zirk, E. Schulze, and T. Bock, "Development and Evaluation of an Assistive Workstation for Cloud Manufacturing in an Aging Society," in *Ambient Assisted Living Advanced Technologies and Societal Change*, 2016.

[150] S. M. Sheweka and N. M. Mohamed, "Green Facades as a New Sustainable Approach towards Climate Change," *Energy Procedia*, pp. 507–520, 2012.

[151] S. Government, "VOI Multipurpose Scooter," [Online]. Available: www.nrf.gov.sg/innovation-enterprise/innovative-projects/urban-solutions-and-sustainability/voi-multipurpose-scooter. [Zugriff am 28 June 2018].

[152] M. Helal, "Transformation of Informal Settlements in Egypt into Productive City Entities by Utilizing and Adapting Advanced Technologies," Munich, Germany, Technical University of Munich, 2016.

[153] K. Lynch, *The Image of the City*, Cambridge, MA, MIT Press, 1975.

[154] T. Bock and T. Linner, *Robot-Oriented Design: Design and Management Tools for the Deployment of Automation and Robotics in Construction*, Cambridge, Cambridge University Press, 2015.

[155] W. Pan, B. Ilhan, and T. Bock, "Process Information Modelling (PIM) for Public Housing Construction Project in Hong Kong," in *Proceedings of Creative Construction Conference 2018 (CCC 2018)*, 2018.

[156] R. Hu, W. Pan, and T. Bock, "A Novel Approach to Develop Vertical City Utilizing Construction Automation and Robotics," in *Proceedings of Creative Construction Conference 2018 (CCC 2018)*, 2018.

[157] T. Linner and T. Bock, "Demografic Change Robotics: Mechatronic Assisted Living and Integrated Robot Technology," in *Introduction to Modern Robotics II*, 2012, pp. 19–46.

[158] R. N. Golden, B. N. Gaynes, R. D. Ekstrom, R. M. Hamer, F. M. Jacobsen, T. Suppes, K. L. Wisner, and C. B. Nemeroff, "The Efficacy of Light Therapy in the Treatment of Mood Disorders: A Review and Meta-Analysis of the Evidence," *The American Journal of Psychiatry*; *Vol. 162, No. 4*, pp. 656–662, 01 April 2005.

[159] M. Braun, S. Gran, O. Kloss, S. Mangold, M. Möres, H. Schulze, M. Schwer, and F. Steffen, "Senioren im Straßenverkehr," *Projektbericht in Zusammenarbeit mit,* 2006.

[160] K. Krämer, "Alt & Mobil: Kompetenzen älterer Verkehrsteilnehmer," *Presseseminar "Senioren im Straßenverkehr". Leipzig,* p. 17, 2004.

[161] T. Linner, B. Ellmann, and T. Bock, "Ubiquitous Life Support Systems for an Ageing Society in Japan," in *Ambient Assisted Living*, Berlin Heidelberg, Springer, 2011, pp. 31–48.

[162] M. Burkhard and K. Michael, "Evaluating Touchscreen Interfaces of Tablet Computers for Elderly People," *Mensch & Computer Workshopband,* 2012.

[163] K. M. Wisdom, S. L. Delp, and E. Kuhl, "Use It or Lose It: Multiscale Skeletal Muscle Adaptation to Mechanical Stimuli," *Biomechanics and Modeling in Mechanobiology*; *Vol.* 14, *No.* 2, pp. 195–215, April 2015.

[164] J. Güttler, T. Linner, C. Georgoulas, and T. Bock, "Development of a Seamless Mobility Chain in the Home Environment," in *Proceedings of the 8th AAL Conference*, Frakfurt, 2015.

[165] Statistische Bundesämter des Bundes und der Länder, "Demografischer Wandel in Deutschland," Heft 1, Statisches Bundesamt, Wiesbaden, 2011.

[166] B. P. B. Mayer, *Die Berliner Altersstudie (BASE): Überblick und Einführung*, Berlin, Akademie Verlag, 1996, pp. 21–54.

[167] G. Doblhammer, R. D. Scholz, and H. Maier, "Month of Birth and Survival to Age 105+: Evidence from the Age Validation Study of German Semi-Supercentenarians," *Experimental Gerontology,* 2005.

[168] J.-M. Robine, A. Cournil, J. Gampe, and J. W. Vaupel, "IDL, the International Database on Longevity," in *Living to 100 and beyond*, Orlando, 2005.

[169] D. Bassily, C. Georgoulas, J. Güttler, T. Linner, and B. T., "Intuitive and Adaptive Robotic Arm Manipulation using the Leap Motion Controller," in *Proceedings of the 45th International Symposium on Robotics (ISR 2014) and the 8th German Conference on Robotics (ROBOTIK 2014)*, Munich, Germany, 2014.

[170] J. Güttler, R. Shah, C. Georgoulas, and T. Bock, "Unobtrusive Tremor Detection and Measurement via Human-Machine Interaction," in *Proceedings of the 5th International Conference on Current and Future Trends of Information and Communication Technologies in Healthcare (ICTH2015)*, Berlin, Germany, 2015.

[171] J. Güttler, C. Georgoulas, and T. Bock, "Adaptive Speed and Sensitivity Configuration of a Robotic Arm with Parallel Health Status Validation via a Gesture-Based Controller Interface," in *Proceedings of the 32nd International Symposium on Automation and Robotics in Construction and Mining*, Oulu, Finland, 2015.

[172] A. Salarian, H. Russmann, C. Wider, P. R. Burkhard, F. J. G. Vingerhoets, and K. Aminian, "Quantification of Tremor and Bradykinesia in Parkinson's Disease Using a Novel Ambulatory Monitoring System," in *IEEE Transactions on Biomedical Engineering*, Vol. 54, No. 2, 2007.

[173] J. Jankovic, "Parkinson's Disease: Clinical Features and Diagnosis," *Journal of Neurology, Neurosurgery & Psychiatry*, Vol. 79, No. 4, pp. 368–376, 2008.

[174] L. Simonsen, M. J. Clarke, L. B. Schonberger, and N. H. Arden, "Pandemic versus Epidemic Influenza Mortality: A Pattern of Changing Age Distribution," *The Journal of Infectious Diseases*, Vol. 178, No. 1, pp. 53–60, 1998.

[175] P. A. Mackowiak, "Physiological Rationale for Suppression of Fever," *Clinical Infectious Diseases*, Vol. 31, No. 5, pp. 185–189, 2000.

[176] A. S. El-Radhi and S. Patel, "An Evaluation of Tympanic Thermometry in a Paediatric Emergency Department," *Emergency Medicine Journal*, Vol. 23, No. 1, pp. 40–41, 2006.

[177] S. Smitz, T. Giagoultsis, W. Dewé, and A. Albert, "Comparison of Rectal and Infrared Ear Temperatures in Older Hospital Inpatients," *Journal of the American Geriatrics Society*, Vol. 48, No. 1, pp. 63–66, 2000.

[178] G. I. Gasim, I. R. Musa, A. M. T., and A. Ishag, "Accuracy of Tympanic Temperature Measurement Using an Infrared Tympanic Membrane Thermometer," *BMC Research Notes*, Vol. 6, No. 1, pp. 1–5, 2013.

[179] M. Dettenkofer and F. Daschner, "Prävention von Infektionen in der Dialyse," in *Praktische Krankenhaushygiene und Umweltschutz*, Berlin Heidelberg, Springer, 1997, pp. 503–518.

[180] J. Güttler, C. Georgoulas, and T. Bock, "Contactless Fever Measurement Based on Thermal Imagery Analysis," in *IEEE Sensors Application*, Catania, 2016.

[181] T. Komensky, M. Jurcisin, K. Ruman, and O. Kovac, "Ultra-Wearable Capacitive Coupled and Common Electrode-Free," in *Annual International Conference of the IEEE Engineering in Medicine and Biology Society*, San Diego, 2012.

[182] A. Steinhage and C. Lauterbach, "SensFloor(R): Ein AAL Sensorsystem für Sicherheit, Homecare und Komfort," in *Ambient Assisted Living - AAL - 1. Deutscher AAL-Kongress mit Ausstellung / Technologien - Anwendungen - Management*, Berlin, 2008.

[183] S. González-Valenzuela, X. Liang, H. Cao, M. Chen, and V. C. Leung, "Body Area Network," in *Autonomous Sensor Networks: Collective Sensing Strategies for Analytical Purposes*, Berlin/Heidelberg, Springer, 2012, pp. 17–38.

[184] J. Alvarez-Lozano, V. Osmani, O. Mayora, M. Frost, J. Bardram, M. Faurholt-Jepsen, and L. V. Kessing, "Tell Me Your Apps and I Will Tell You Your Mood: Correlation of Apps Usage with Bipolar Disorder State," in *Proceedings of the 7th International Conference on PErvasive Technologies Related to Assistive Environments*, New York, 2014.

[185] M. R. Bice, J. W. Ball, and S. McClaran, "Technology and Physical Activity Motivation," *International Journal of Sport and Exercise Psychology*, pp. 1–10, 2015.

[186] A. Ahtinen, M. Isomursu, S. Ramiah, and J. Blom, "Advise, Acknowledge, Grow and Engage: Design Principles for a Mobile Wellness Application to Support Physical Activity," *International Journal of Mobile Human Computer Interaction*, Vol. 5, No. 4, pp. 20–55, 2013.

[187] E. H. Conrow, "Estimating Technology Readiness Level Coefficients," *Jouernal of Spacecraft and Rockets*, Vol. 48, No. 1, pp. 146–152, 2011.

[188] Lufthansa Technik, [Online]. Available: www.lufthansa-technik.com/innovation-projects. [Zugriff am 18 10 2017].

[189] C. Fernandez-Andres, A. Iborra, B. Alvarez, J. A. Pastor, P. Sanchez, J. M. Fernandez-Merono, and N. Ortega, "Ship Shape in Europe: Cooperative Robots in the Ship Repair Industry," *IEEE Robotics & Automation Magazine*, Vol. 12, No. 3, pp. 65–77, 2005.

[190] "Statoil Robotic Lab," [Online]. Available: https://robotnor.no/expertise/lab-facilities/statoil-robotics-lab/. [Zugriff am 08 12 2017].

[191] F. G. Mangano, B. Cirotti, R. L. Sammons, and C. Mangano, "Custom-Made, Root-Analogue Direct Laser Metal Forming Implant: A Case Report," *Lasers in Medical Science*, Vol. 27, No. 6, pp. 1241–1245, 2012.

[192] S. P. Bhumkar, V. V. Deotare, and R. V. Babar, "Intelligent Car System for Accident Prevention Using ARM-7," *International Journal of Emerging Technology and Advanced Engineering*, Vol. 2, No. 4, pp. 527–531, 2012.

[193] W.-B. Horng, C.-Y. Chen, C. Yi, and C.-H. Fan, "Driver Fatigue Detection Based on Eye Tracking and Dynamic Template Matching," in *Proceedings of the 2004 IEEE International Conference on Networking, Sensing & Control*, Taipei, 2004.

[194] M. Santamouris, T. Bock, S. Isaac, A. L. Pisello, R. Gupta, M. Kyprianou-Dracou, D. Kolokotsa, P. Perani, S. Koehler, S. Chadiarakou, F. M. Montagnino, M. Isaac, B. Jehl, G. L. Continanza, M. Sammoutis, and O. Daggett, *Achieving Near Zero and Positive Energy Settlements in Europe Using Advanced Energy Technology*, Horizon 2020-EE-2015-1-PPP, 2015.

Index